Arthritis

WHAT EXERCISES WORK

ALSO BY DAVA SOBEL AND ARTHUR C. KLEIN

Arthritis: What Works

Backache Relief

Arthritis

WHAT EXERCISES WORK

Dava Sobel &

Arthur C. Klein

Illustrations by John Dickinson

St. Martin's Press   New York

ARTHRITIS: WHAT EXERCISES WORK. Copyright © 1993 by Dava Sobel and Arthur C. Klein. All rights reserved. Printed in the United States of America. No part of this book may be used or reproduced in any manner whatsoever without written permission except in the case of brief quotations embodied in critical articles or reviews. For information, address St. Martin's Press, 175 Fifth Avenue, New York, N.Y. 10010.

Editor: Jared Kieling
Production Editor: Eric C. Meyer
Copyedited by Carla Sommerstien
Design by Robin Hessel Hoffmann

Library of Congress Cataloging-in-Publication Data

Sobel, Dava.
    Arthritis: what exercises work / Dava Sobel and Arthur C. Klein; foreword by John Bland.
      p.   cm.
    ISBN 0-312-09743-3
    1. Arthritis—Exercise therapy.   I. Klein, Arthur C.   II. Title.
RC933.S6148   1993
616.7'22062—dc20   93-26697
                                                  CIP

Books are available in quantity for promotional or premium use. Write to Director of Special Sales, St. Martin's Press, 175 Fifth Avenue, New York, N.Y. 10010, for information on discounts and terms, or call toll-free (800) 221-7945. In New York, call (212) 674-5151 (ext. 645).

CONTENTS

PART THREE
Aerobic Fitness Exercises for Arthritis — 39

PART FOUR
Exercising Away Pain from Head to Toe — 65

PART FIVE
Exercising under Special Circumstances — 181

FOREWORD

When Dava Sobel and Arthur Klein first asked me to write a foreword to *Arthritis: What Exercises Work,* I was a little less than enthusiastic. I wondered whether I should accept their invitation, for I suspected the book might be "just another patient care book," whereas I have been deeply involved in rheumatology (the subspecialty of medicine that concentrates on all forms of arthritis) for forty years. As it turned out, I was honored, delighted, and educated in reading—indeed *studying*—the manuscript. I believe that this book and its predecessor, *Arthritis: What Works,* are practical, scientifically sound, well written, and instantly comprehensible. Together, they offer the best advice available today in overall management of the two most widespread forms of arthritis, rheumatoid arthritis and osteoarthritis.

Arthritis: What Exercises Work deals with one of the most important and significant aspects of the management of these two diseases. Exercise is very commonly prescribed for arthritis, but that's about as far as it all too frequently goes. In other words, doctors give patients too little detail or instruction, with few illustrations, and no precise direction. Yet many of the most troublesome and disabling aspects of both rheumatoid arthritis and osteoarthritis are due to lack of exercise!

A joint that is immobilized initiates a series of changes that result in total destruction of the joint within about four months. This occurs even in the absence of disease—by dint of immobilization alone. Adhesions begin to appear in the joint, a strange tissue grows over the surface of the cartilage, and tears occur where tendons are inserted in bone. New planes of motion contrary to normal anatomical planes appear, followed by enzymatic degradation of the tissues. Ligaments become lax, losing their tensile strength. The cartilage that caps the ends of bones, and which is normally four times more slippery than Teflon, loses that slipperiness and becomes perforated by ulcers.

Many of the changes that occur in the joints of people with rheumatoid arthritis and osteoarthritis are assumed to be caused by a disease process, when in fact they are often a consequence of relative immobility. These findings underscore the enormous importance of exercise in the fight against arthritis. I always counsel my patients to exercise to their point of tolerance.

My advice to you, the reader, is the same. You should realize that immobility will set off the destructive set of events I outlined above in just a few weeks. After four or five months, such degeneration may be quite well along, so that even if you initiate a program of vigorous exercise, you may have to wait up to a year for the joint's normal motion to return. Therefore, I say, prevention is the order of the day.

Exercise exerts a very favorable influence on the immunological system, affecting the production of white blood cells, lymphocytes and leukocytes, as well as the whole spectrum of antibodies against various viruses and bacteria. A protective agent called interferon is induced by brisk exercise. There is even evidence that people who are exercising significantly lower their risk of cancer. Exercising also reduces obesity.

Actively exercising to the best of your ability helps you discover your own fountain of youth. Do not heed the warning that because you have a disease you should rest more and more, and not stretch yourself at all. That would be the worst thing you could do.

Stretching, described in the book, is of major importance as a prelude to walking and as a regular habit to maintain healthy ligaments, muscles, bones, joints, and tendons. A complete stretching program would require approximately ten to fifteen minutes a day. It is wise to stretch before and after a walk, to help you maintain optimum balance, and avoid stumbling and falls.

Warm up before you exercise, and cool down afterward with some postexercise stretching.

Walking, which almost everyone with rheumatoid arthritis or osteoarthritis can do to some degree, is of extreme importance as an integral, essential part of a program of disease management. I've come to use the term "walk the walk" when urging my patients to carry themselves proudly, and to remember that self-confidence is the most important mental ingredient for success in arthritis management. The way you walk and move can strongly influence the way you think and feel. If your body is down, your thoughts and feeling will be down. If your body is up, your thoughts and feelings will be up, too.

Walking the walk means holding your head high and your chin up, while keeping your eyes forward, shoulders back, and arms swinging to the bounce in your step. It is difficult to walk the walk and say things like "I'm awful," "I hurt," or "I can't do this." Rather, a person who walks the walk says, "I am confident in my ability," "I know how to handle pressure," and "I'm going to practice walking the walk by being aware of how I carry myself."

When you focus on making positive physical changes, as this book shows you, you'll feel more positive and energetic.

To exercise, and especially to walk, is to induce the synthesis and release of a set of hormones called endorphins produced in the brain and the spinal cord. These normal, morphinelike substances actually diminish the perception of pain. Equally, or perhaps more important, is the fact that walking generates a sense of self-esteem, with increased optimism and decreased anxiety. Thus, walking confers both a physical and an intellectual appreciation of self-worth.

Increasing self-confidence not only makes you feel better physically and psychologically, but also improves sexual appetite and performance. You will look better and feel younger. You will grow tougher and more content. Best of all, you can say to yourself, "I set out to do it, and I did it."

Until recently, the question of how intensely one must exercise was unresolved. Taking a hint from a well-known fable, we can see that although the tortoise and the hare travel at different paces, the tortoise is the less anxious. You don't have to work up to a sweat to experience the stress-relieving and tissue-saving benefits of exercise. The evidence now is that walking, even at a slow pace, can induce the mechanisms in the body (arthritis or no arthritis!) that elevate mood, relieve anxiety, and improve one's overall self-esteem. Joint stiffness is reduced. Swelling tends to gradually disappear with regular walking. The prevention of bone loss is another benefit of walking.

As the authors of this book point out, walking is one of the few exercises to which age and physical condition usually pose no barriers.

I also consider it of great importance to exercise your brain. By that, I mean I encourage you to practice memory methods, remain with the times, read, study, and be all you can be. I know I still see myself as an underachiever. I haven't run as fast as I can, I haven't walked as fast as I can, I haven't written as well as I can. Not yet! I can still strive to do better. And so can you. Regardless of the presence of a chronic disease—or anything else—you are capable of improved physical and intellectual performance. This book will help you achieve them.

—John H. Bland, M.D.
Professor of Medicine,
University of Vermont
College of Medicine

INTRODUCTION

How Arthritis: What Exercises
Work *came to be*

The nationwide survey we conducted for our previous book, *Arthritis: What Works*, revealed that exercise is the single best treatment for the pain and disability of arthritis. Not only does exercise often succeed where drugs, braces, and surgery have failed to relieve pain, but exercise can also help restore the normal appearance and full function of the joints.

Having heard hundreds of our 1,051 Arthritis Survey participants attest to the value of proper exercise, we included two chapters of exercise advice in *Arthritis: What Works*, which has sold over 400,000 copies since its publication in 1989, thus becoming the best-selling hardcover arthritis self-help guide in its field.

What did our readers think about our two chapters of exercise advice? Frankly, they loved it—but they wanted more. They wanted more of the latest information about exercises recommended for overall fitness. They wanted more specific movements devised to improve flexibility. They wanted proven, effective activities for increasing strength while minimizing pain.

In short, they wanted a new guide! One completely devoted to exercise, filled with practical advice and with drawings that make the step-by-step instructions easy to follow.

They wanted the ultimate arthritis exercise guide. One that could dramatically change their lives. This has been our goal in writing *Arthritis: What Exercises Work.*

The book you have in your hands fully explores the types of exercise that benefit people with arthritis. These range from overall aerobic activities, through strengthening (isometric and isotonic) exercises, to range-of-motion workouts that increase the mobility of each individual joint.

Most of the exercises in this book were derived from our original survey participants' experiences, and were then reviewed and refined with the help of two exercise experts, Dr. Willibald Nagler and Dr. Irene von Estorff of the Department of Physical Medicine and Rehabilitation at The New York Hospital–Cornell Medical Center in New York City. The book also contains additional exercises contributed recently by readers who found the book helpful and wrote to us to share their positive experiences with exercise.

This book contains:

- Self-evaluation checklists to help you determine a safe level of activity and set reasonable exercise goals
- Strategies for devising your own individually tailored beginner's exercise program
- Explanations of the different types of exercises, with directions on how to combine them for maximum benefit

- Instructions on how to increase your activity levels over time
- Guidelines for modifying your exercise regimen during an arthritis flare-up or when specific joints become inflamed and swollen
- Suggestions on how to integrate exercise routines into your everyday activities
- Tips on how to make simple exercise equipment with materials you can find around your house, and
- Advice from others with arthritis on how to get motivated to start an exercise program. (You needn't worry about keeping motivation high once you get rolling. Your own pain relief and increased activity will surely keep you going then!)

Part 1, "The Life-Enhancing Value of Exercise for Arthritis," will guide you in constructing your own exercise program from the book's large assortment of suggested activites. Part 2, "Mental Gymnastics," covers relaxation techniques that will complement your exercise regimen, as well as give you tips on how to warm up and cool down. The aerobic exercises—such as walking, swimming, cycling, and dancing—are discussed in part 3, "Aerobic Fitness Exercises for Arthritis." Stretching and strengthening exercises appear in part 4, "Exercising Away Pain from Head to Toe"; individual exercises are grouped into chapters by joint—from neck and jaw to ankles and feet. In part 5, "Exercising under Special Circumstances," you'll find advice on particular situations—including safe exercise during a flare-up, precautions for pre- and postsurgery exercise routines, and ways to modify arthritis exercise to accommodate other health problems.

We hope you will show this book to your doctor, physical therapists, or exercise instructor. We anticipate that these professionals will welcome the information it contains, especially if they themselves have not had detailed instruction in prescribing exercise for arthritis.

Indeed, many of our original survey participants said that they had been told to exercise—but were never told how!—presumably because their doctors didn't know or didn't have time to explain. Some were given the wrong exercises—and made to suffer needlessly—by practitioners who should have known better.

This book combines documented-safe exercises with cookbook-style directions and illustrations, based on the accumulated experience of many people with physical problems similar to yours—people who understand firsthand the challenge and the value of regular exercise in the treatment of arthritis.

We encourage you to begin at once by starting to move more today. Why wait until you feel better to begin, when beginning to exercise can help you to feel better now? Ready? Let's proceed together. We want to help you every step of the way!

Arthritis

WHAT EXERCISES WORK

The Life-Enhancing Value of Exercise for Arthritis

> *The weakest and oldest among us can become some sort of athlete, but only the strongest can survive as spectators, only the hardiest can withstand the perils of inertia, inactivity, and immobility.*
>
> —Drs. J. H. Bland and S. M. Cooper
> from *Seminars in Arthritis and Rheumatism*

CHAPTER 1

The Miracle "Drug" That You Can Give Yourself

What to expect from your own arthritis exercise program

Truly, the value of exercise in fighting arthritis cannot be overstated. Its effectiveness is demonstrated beyond question, both in our Arthritis Survey results and in numerous medical studies conducted at hospitals. Rest, which was long touted as the best treatment for arthritis, has proved to be a poor and often destructive substitute for activity.

As we discovered while doing research for our previous book, *Arthritis: What Works*, exercise helped ninety-five percent of those Arthritis Survey participants who tried it. No other approach to arthritis—no drug, no surgical procedure—matches exercise for high rates of improvement. Nor can any other treatment modality boast exercise's low risk of serious complications or unpleasant side effects.

Exercise figures in every good comprehensive treatment plan for arthritis. It is the all-purpose adjunct therapy for individuals at every stage of ability and disability. *Whatever else people do for their arthritis, they do better if they exercise as well.*

Many problems that are usually attributed to arthritis itself, such as poor posture and hesitant gait, are really the result of inactivity. Exercise is the key to better body mechanics—to feeling and doing better.

According to our nationwide study, the chief benefits that you stand to gain from exercise are (1) increased flexibility of your affected joints, and (2) pain relief. Many Arthritis Survey participants also told us that regular exercise (3) improved their general health by lowering high blood pressure and cholesterol levels, and even (4) helped those with diabetes to gain better control over their blood-sugar levels.

In addition to these results, or perhaps in part because of them, our respondents also credited exercise with (5) lifting their spirits, (6) helping them fight stress, (7) giving them more energy during the day, and (8) ensuring better sleep at night. Thus, it (9) improved the overall quality of their lives.

Sounds like a miracle drug—and it is.

Arguments in favor of exercise only increase as one gets older. Among individuals between the ages of fifty-five and eighty-eight, a recent study at Scripps College revealed, regular exercise (10) rendered people better able to reason, remember, and solve problems. In Dallas, investigations with thousands of men and women at The Institute for Aerobics Research and the Cooper Clinic showed that even moderate exercise would (11) significantly reduce a person's chance of dying of heart disease or cancer.

Since exercise can also help keep weight in check, it can (12) retard or altogether prevent the development of arthritis in certain joints. A very encouraging study supported by the National Institutes of Health showed that overweight women who drop roughly a pound a year for ten years can often avoid osteoarthritis of the knee.

The motion of exercise nourishes the joints: with motion, fluids are squeezed in and out of the joint space, delivering nourishment to the cartilage, getting rid of waste products. Without motion, this vital exchange cannot take place. The cartilage covering the ends of the bones where they meet has no blood supply of its own. The only way for the cartilage to take in needed nutrients and oxygen is via the motion of the joint. (In osteoarthritis, the cartilage is particularly vulnerable to destruction.)

We trust that if you've read this far, you're fairly well convinced that you want to begin an exercise program. Great. Now the question is: What kind of exercise should you do?

Arthritis exercise comes in three prescription strengths:

- *Aerobic activities,* such as walking and swimming, that build stamina and boost cardiovascular fitness
- *Stretching, or "range of motion" exercises,* such as leg raises and finger curls, that keep the joints mobile
- *Strengthening exercises,* including lifting light weights, that prevent muscle atrophy.

Each type plays a role in maintaining and improving your overall flexibility, as well as in preventing the deformities that arthritis can cause.

This book offers instructions in all three types of arthritis exercise. Please don't be discouraged by the range of options available to you. No one is expected to work through all the maneuvers at any one time. Rather, we hope you'll use the book the way you'd consult a menu at a restaurant: you choose what suits you from the many available possibilities. The rest of part 1, like a helpful waiter, provides explanations, suggestions, and sample combinations.

Aerobic exercises tend to be everyone's favorites because they are intrinsically enjoyable, or can be made that way. Many of them can be done in the company of others, and therefore provide opportunities for pleasant social contacts. Walking is our favorite aerobic exercise since it is safe and effective, and can be done virtually anywhere. Walking can be easily adapted to your level of fitness by adjusting the speed and duration of the activity. For example, some people can put their sneakers on every day, and walk at a rapid clip for forty-five minutes to an hour, covering as much ground as three or four miles. Less-fit beginners will want to start off slowly, with the goal of doing just a little bit more walking than they've been used to. If you're starting from zero, you might begin with a walk from one room to another right in your own home, or around the block once or twice.

Aerobic exercise will increase your general level of fitness and endurance over time. It will also give you relief from much of your pain and stiffness by increasing the blood flow to your affected joints and muscles. To guarantee the flexibility of individual joints, however, you need range-of-motion exercises that stretch every single joint, every day. You will no doubt want to concentrate on those joints that are most in need of attention because they ache or fail you in your regular activities. You may want to help yourself further by giving some exercise attention to your smoothly functioning joints as well, to ensure that they will *continue* to function dependably. Don't worry about doing this extra work right away, however, especially at the outset, when you can easily get overwhelmed by a program that is too time-consuming or confusing.

The strengthening exercises that build up your muscles give your joints the best possible protection from injury and deformity. Strengthening exercises may be isotonic or isometric. The *isotonic* ones involve motion against resistance. For example, when you raise and lower your arm hefting a can of tomatoes, the can's weight provides the resistance that makes your arm work hard and get strong. (The same movement without the can would be a range-of-motion stretch.) The *isometric* exercises involve no movement of the joint, just force

6

against resistance. Pushing against a wall, for example, is another way to strengthen your arm. The wall never moves, of course, but your muscles are still working. The lack of motion makes such exercises do-able even on days when your joints hurt too much to engage in isotonic activity. Isometric exercises promise considerable gains in strength and pain relief, but the gains disappear quickly if you drop the exercises.

Now that you know the general types of exercises you will be doing, it's time to assess your own abilities and preferences in order to determine your exercise prescription. Please turn to chapter 2, and get a pen or pencil ready to answer some questions about yourself.

CHAPTER 2

Only You Can Write the Right Exercise Prescription

How to gauge your physical condition

and exercise readiness

Many medical and nonmedical practitioners, from rheumatologists to yoga instructors, advise exercise, but not all of them can prescribe it effectively. Our aim in this chapter is to guide you to the best possible exercise help—and also to encourage you to become your own reliable expert in the matter of arthritis exercise.

The practitioners who enjoy the most success in teaching beneficial exercise, according to our research, are physical therapists with a special interest in arthritis. These individuals provide a variety of treatments that temporarily relieve arthritis pain, such as ultrasound, diathermy, and massage, but they get their best long-term results by devising personally tailored exercise programs and by encouraging people in their care to exercise daily. Physical therapists, unfortunately, are in short supply: according to some estimates, people with arthritis outnumber physical therapists by more than one thousand to one.

Although physical therapists rarely failed to help our Arthritis Survey participants in their care, a few did cause harm by being incompetent or insensitive. If you feel the advice or the treatments you get from a physical therapist are not helping—or worse, are *harming*—you, then stop them immediately.

Another potentially excellent source of exercise advice is your doctor. But if he or she has not yet recommended exercise, then we urge you to raise the subject as soon as possible. Please discuss your exercise plans on your very next visit to the doctor's office—and take this book along with you to break the ice.

If your doctor resists the idea of exercise, which is unlikely, then please seek a second medical opinion. The types of doctors who provided the most help to our Arthritis Survey participants—and the best exercise advice—were rheumatologists (arthritis specialists), orthopedists (also called orthopedic surgeons), and physiatrists (doctors of physical medicine and rehabilitation).

Exercise instructors at local gyms and fitness centers also helped many of our Arthritis Survey participants. If you seek advice from one of these experts, however, please make certain that the instructor understands the special needs of people who have arthritis, and has experience working with them.

Ultimately, you will become your own best exercise expert, because only you can judge the difficulty of any given maneuver, the pain it causes you during or after your exercise session, the improvement it brings to your condition, and the change in your strength and endurance over time.

We provide a great many step-by-step instructions in this book, because we know how daunting it can be to undertake a new self-treatment. You may rely heavily on the instructions at first, until you master the material you need to pursue your own exercise prescription. Soon you will be using it only occasionally, to refresh your memory or give you ideas for more advanced routines.

Osteoarthritis vs. Rheumatoid Arthritis

The exercises in this book are intended for people who have either osteoarthritis or rheumatoid arthritis, which are the two most common forms of arthritis. They differ from each other in their cause and effect.

Osteoarthritis is a "wear and tear" condition in which the cartilage protecting the ends of the bones flakes off, leaving rough edges and preventing the joints from functioning smoothly. Most often, the joints affected by osteoarthritis are the "weight-bearing" joints, especially the knees, hips, back, and neck. It is not uncommon for disabilities to make themselves felt on one side of the body and not the other, so that the left knee is extremely stiff and painful while the right knee feels fine.

Rheumatoid arthritis is an autoimmune disease, in which the body's own agents attack the tissues of the joints, often making them feel hot and swollen. The joints most commonly affected by rheumatoid arthritis are the hands, wrists, ankles, and feet, and the pain tends to be symmetrical on both sides of the body.

All the participants in our Arthritis Survey had received a diagnosis of either osteoarthritis, rheumatoid arthritis, or both. In general, rheumatoid arthritis tends to set in at a younger age, and to grow alternately better and worse for no apparent reason over the course of time. People with rheumatoid arthritis also experience fatigue that limits their stamina, although they can increase their stamina through exercise.

Exercise is beneficial for everyone with arthritis, regardless of type. What differentiates your exercise program from someone else's will have more to do with your level of fitness and the number of affected joints than with the form of arthritis you have.

Know Your Limits—And Potential

Exercise programs differ because people differ so vastly in their abilities and needs. Start to assess your basic exercise level with the following simple quiz. Circle one answer to each question.

QUIZ 1: EXERCISE READINESS

I consider myself:
- (1) very active
- (2) moderately active
- (3) inactive by choice—a "couch potato"
- (4) inactive because of pain or disability

When I get up in the morning, I feel:
- (1) hardly any pain or stiffness
- (2) a fair amount of pain and stiffness that lasts up to twenty minutes
- (3) pain and stiffness that persists for an hour or longer
- (4) severe pain and stiffness that seems never to go away completely

As I go through the day, I find that I:
  (1) can keep up my normal activities pretty comfortably, at work and/or at home
  (2) manage well but need to rest at least once during the day
  (3) need to modify the way I do things and need to rest periodically, but still manage on my own
  (4) need help to do most things

My experience with exercise in general, and arthritis exercise in particular, is:
  (1) extensive
  (2) moderate
  (3) limited
  (4) nonexistent

My age is:
  (1) forty or younger
  (2) forty-one to fifty-five
  (3) fifty-six to sixty-five
  (4) over sixty-five

Now we'd like you to place yourself in one of four categories, depending on the way you answered the above questions. Look at the numbers of the answers you circled. If you circled all ones, for example, or mostly ones, then you can begin with a Level 1 exercise program, which is quite physically demanding. Likewise, if you circled all twos, then begin with a Level 2 program, which is a little less taxing. If you circled some twos and some threes, begin with the Level 3 for safety's sake. (You can always advance yourself more quickly later if you find the Level 3 is too simple for you.) If you skipped around with your answers, from one to four, then the safest course for you is to begin with a Level 4 program, then modify it accordingly.

The next quiz will help you assess the condition of your joints, so that you can determine the areas that need the most attention in your exercise program. No doubt you have several affected joints, and some are more painful than others. Thus, your personal exercise routine might include very gentle motions for your fingers, for example, but more vigorous shoulder and elbow movements.

QUIZ 2: JOINT CONDITION

Grade each of your joints according to the following scale:

1 = little or no pain, good range of motion

2 = moderate pain, adequate range of motion

3 = extreme pain, very limited range of motion

4 = inflamed (hot and swollen)

R = surgically replaced joint, painful or painfree, at any level of mobility

Jaw _____	Back _____
Neck _____	Hips _____
Shoulders _____	Knees _____
Elbows _____	Ankles _____
Wrists _____	Feet/Toes _____
Hands/Fingers _____	

As in the Exercise Readiness quiz, the grades you give yourself determine the level of activity for each joint. You can then select the relevant stretching and strengthening exercises keyed to your level, knowing you will be able to perform them safely.

If you have a surgically implanted replacement joint, please consult your surgeon before attempting any of the exercises recommended for that part of your body. When selecting aerobic exercise, remember that certain precautions apply to artificial hips and knees, and you need to respect these if you want the joint to last as long as possible.

Every exercise program includes all three types of exercises: 1) aerobic conditioning that has become so highly regarded for its beneficial effect on the heart and lungs, 2) range-of-motion exercises that stretch each individual joint to the fullest extent possible, and 3) strengthening exercises that build up muscle to give the joints strong support. Even the simplest program will combine all three types for best results, because each one complements the other.

Aerobic exercise will benefit your heart and lungs, and relieve pain and stiffness by improving the blood circulation throughout your body. When you read the chapters on the various forms of aerobic exercise in part 3, just select the one that appeals to you most. Feel free to cross train by combining aerobic activities, or pursuing different ones on different days. You may enjoy your exercise program more if you swim three days a week and walk four, for example, or ride a bicycle in the summer and walk through shopping malls in the winter. These activities are easily tailored to your time and tastes. Many people find that variation is the spice that keeps motivation cooking.

When you begin to select range-of-motion and strengthening exercises, you'll want to focus on the joints that hurt, function poorly, or appear obviously affected by arthritic changes. Your other joints can also be put through their paces each day, as a preventive measure—quickly and easily after exercising the problem joints.

You can gauge whether you're doing just the right amount or going too far by the way you feel after you exercise. Pain is a reliable measure of joint strain and muscle overuse. Don't be too alarmed if you feel some discomfort for up to about one hour after your initial workout. If you do the same amount the next day, you should feel less discomfort, and even that will be short-lived. However, if you are considerably sore, or the soreness lasts beyond the one-hour point, your body is telling you to cut back. Please heed the advice.

You can use the guidelines in the next chapter to assemble your own individualized exercise routine, and then fine-tune it as you grow stronger and more flexible. Remember, you don't have to stop there—you can keep modifying your regimen indefinitely, to meet your changing needs. As you become expert in judging the motions that work best for you, you may even want to create your own exercises, combining them with the ones offered here, and devising creative strategies for working exercise into your schedule every day, wherever you are, whatever else you may be doing. Then you'll have mastered your exercise prescription and dosage schedule.

To hasten that day, let's begin to assemble your individually tailored program right now by consulting the advice in chapter 3.

CHAPTER 3

How to Develop a Tailor-Made Exercise Routine

How to combine the three types of exercise into an arthritis exercise program that works for you

Now that you know the kinds of exercise you need, the level of exercise you can safely attempt, and the specific joints that you will emphasize in your daily routine, you can assemble your own exercise program.

It's easier than you think. All you have to do is consult the sample routines laid out beginning on page 18, and then use the blank forms on the following pages to construct your own.

Let's suppose, for example, that you are quite limited by pain, have no significant experience with exercise, and feel too tired to attempt much that is novel or challenging. Your first exercise routine can be one that you carry out in bed, before you even get up to face the day. (In fact, you'll probably find that going through the routine gets you ready—and raring—to start the day!)

outine 1 (Level 4: In-Bed)

Start with the exercise preparation in chapter 4 and the deep breathing and relaxation exercises in chapter 5.

Slowly and gently proceed through the range-of-motion exercises listed below. (Each one is explained step-by-step in chapters 11–19, and the numbers in parentheses after each exercise name tell you where to find it.) At this point, you need not worry about repeating the movements any set number of times. Just see how it feels to stretch your body.

A-E-I-O-U Shout (p.68)
Left-Right (p.72)
Shoulder Shrug (p.69, 76)
Swinging Pendulum (p.76)
Elbow Limber-up (p.100)
Elbow Twist (p.100)
Wrist Assist (p.106)
Wrist Twist (p.108)
Wrist Rotator (p.107)
Finger Spread (p.115)
Okay All Around (p.116)
Pelvic Tilt (p.130)
Knee-to-Chest (p.128)
Leg Spread (p.142)
Leg Roll (p.142)
Straight Leg-ups (p.144)
Liftbacks (p.150)
Knee Push (p.158)
Ankle Twist (p.170)
Foot Circles (p.171)
Toe Curls (p.171)

At first, you may achieve only rough approximations of the movements as they are described. Be patient with yourself. Improvement comes with practice, and you have the rest of your life to perfect your form. If any movements seem wrong for you, however, or cause you sudden pain, then by all means stop them or modify them to suit you.

Later in the day, perhaps after a rest period, repeat the sequence outlined above, and add to it these strengthening exercises:

Bed Head (p.69)
Bodybuilder (p.82) [This *can* be done lying down.]
Alternate Elbow Builder (p.103)
Praying Hands (p.112)
Finger Push-ups (p.118)
Squeeze Play (p.125)
Bent-Knee Sit-ups (p.132)
The Squeeze (p.152)
Knee Press (p.158)
Toe Helper (p.171)

Warning: Be especially gentle with any joint that is hot and swollen. Although it helps to move even inflamed joints through their range of motion, it hurts to do any more. Too much motion can actually cut off the blood circulation to an actively inflamed joint. This is the one case where rest takes precedence over motion. Do very little with your inflamed joints until the flare-up passes. (See chapter 20 for more information about exercise and arthritis flare-ups.)

For your aerobic exercise, try walking (see chapter 6). At first, you may not get true aerobic benefit from the activity, as it's unlikely you'll be able to walk quickly enough to do so. Just concentrate on walking a little farther each day and a little more vigorously than you did the day before.

No doubt you will feel some muscle fatigue in the aftermath of these exercises. That's only natural, and the feeling will gradually disappear as you become more accustomed to the movements. But persistent pain that lasts for more than one hour is different: it's a danger sign of joint overuse. Be kind to yourself: do less the next time. You're better off building up slowly rather than rushing things and suffering a setback.

As you become accustomed to exercising, you can pay more attention to the number of repetitions of each movement. You started with one, and can gradually build up to three or five, then ten, and eventually as many as thirty.

Sample Routine 2 (Level 2: Moderately Active)

You, too, can begin with the part 2 Preparation and Relaxation exercises. You could also use the first sample routine as a morning stretch, even though you are probably capable of more strenuous activity.

Take your pick of the aerobic activities in part 3, and try to pursue one of them for forty-five minutes, at least three times a week. You may vary the activities if you like, so that you walk twice a week, for example, and ride a bicycle twice.

Here is a suggested list of range-of-motion exercises, each of which you can probably repeat three times. But be careful not to push through pain, and if pain following exercise persists for more than one hour, cut back on the number of repetitions. When you can do these easily, you can add more repetitions.

A-E-I-O-U Shout (p.68)
Yes-No (p.70)
Head Roll (p.70)
Shoulder Roll (p.77)
Butterfly Stretch (p.78)
Crisscross (p.84)
Wing Tuck (p.98)
Chop Wood (p.101)

Wrist Twist (p.108)
Wrist Rotator (p.107)
Finger Lifts (p.115)
Typist's Warm-up (p.115)
Pelvic Tilt (p.130)
Knee Drops (p.132)
Leg Lifts (p.150)
Liftbacks (p.150)
Knee to Chest Plus (p.156)
Knee Kicks (p.159)
Foot Circles (p.171)
Soft Shoe (p.172)

Feel free to add to the list if you want to give extra attention to specific joints that need more exercise.

Here are some isometric and isotonic exercises to strengthen your muscles:

Neck Push (p.73,158)
Wallflower (p.89)
Push-offs (p.92)
Elbow Builder (p.103)
Wrist Rise (p.110)
Finger Skids (p.124)
Sit-downs (p.134)
Hip Strengthener (p.152)
Ballet Bends (p.162)
Ankle Builder (p.178)

You can use the following forms to record your own exercise plan, and then keep track of additions and changes. This is a good way to mark your progress and to troubleshoot for the causes of later soreness, but if it seems like too much paper work for you, by all means just move on to the next chapter and start moving.

ARTHRITIS EXERCISE PROGRESS CHART

Week #   Day #

Aerobic activity ——————   Length of time ——————

Range of Motion Exercises

Joint	Exercise #	Number of Repetitions
———————	———————	———————————
———————	———————	———————————
———————	———————	———————————
———————	———————	———————————
———————	———————	———————————
———————	———————	———————————
———————	———————	———————————
———————	———————	———————————
———————	———————	———————————
———————	———————	———————————
———————	———————	———————————
———————	———————	———————————
———————	———————	———————————

ARTHRITIS EXERCISE PROGRESS CHART

Week #   Day #

Aerobic activity _____   Length of time _____

Stretching and Strengthening Exercises

Joint	Exercise #	Number of Repetitions

P A R T
T W O

Mental Gymnastics

> *There are many misconceptions regarding meditation. A common one is that the process of meditation is austere. Another is that meditation is boring. Sometimes meditating is viewed as passive, a withdrawal from the world, for wimps, not productive people. Exercise, in contrast, is seen as active, macho, getting out there and really* doing *something.*
>
> —Dean Ornish, M.D.

CHAPTER 4

Preparation for Exercise

How to get yourself mentally and physically ready to begin your arthritis exercise program

The commitment you're making to give yourself the benefit of regular exercise is one of the most important steps you can take to improve your arthritis. It's like turning over a new leaf, or making a New Year's resolution. Now, while you're feeling motivated and confident, is the time to build in safeguards for your exercise program.

You can make the program inviting and therefore effective by the way you set it up and go about it. The right music played in the background, for example, can increase the pleasure you derive from your exercise period, and help to make you feel good about the time spent exercising, even before the activity becomes its own reward.

Here are some reminders of the promises exercise can fulfill:

Pain relief
Greater stamina
Increased range of motion
Added strength
Improved joint function
Extra energy
Heightened self-sufficiency
Brighter outlook
Better sleep
Normalized blood pressure and cholesterol levels
Loss of excess weight

Starting an exercise program is a way of taking control of your future. By exercising, you give your body the best possible chance of beating the odds arthritis has stacked against you. Planning and sticking to an exercise regimen shows you care about yourself. Your actions prove that you refuse to give in to the feelings of helplessness and depression that often accompany arthritis.

Setting the Stage

You may do your first exercises of the day in bed, as part of the routine that helps you arise feeling limber. Later on in the day you'll probably need to choose a different setting for your aerobic, stretching, and strengthening exercises. The time and place are important determinants of success.

You may have noticed a particular hour in your daily routine when you seem to have more than your usual vim and vigor—and the least possible pain. People with rheumatoid arthritis frequently find that their pain tends to be worse in the mornings, and so prefer to exercise in the afternoons. In contrast, people with osteoarthritis tend to feel best in the morning, and then notice an increase in pain as the day progresses.

If you're free to exercise at your peak-energy time, by all means seize the moment. If not, then look for an opportunity when you can rest for fifteen or twenty minutes before starting to exercise. A catnap or brief period of quiet meditation may recapture some of the bounce and enthusiasm that will smoothe your way.

If you take pain medications, please be mindful of how you schedule the timing of your drug prescription and your exercise prescription. The two don't really mix well. If you begin to exercise at the moment your pain medication reaches its peak of power, your body may miss important pain messages. You may be unable to sense the twinges that would normally signal you to abandon an activity beyond your ability. You want to feel as comfortable as possible when you begin exercising, but not so comfortable as to be oblivious to danger.

Warming Up

Preheating your muscles for exercise helps you avoid strain. Many people think of warm-ups as activities in themselves, such as stretching the legs before running. However, there are safe, effective warm-up techniques that can *precede* even the simplest actions.

In bed, for example, sleeping under an electric blanket or down comforter gets your whole body toasty. This warmth is the ideal prelude for an in-bed exercise routine.

Later in the day, you may warm up for an exercise period by dressing in extra layers of clothing, or by taking a warm bath or shower, followed by an application of liniment. This form of passive warm-up is all that is needed for most stretching and strengthening exercises. In fact, numerous exercises can actually be done while you are lying in a warm tub or standing under a hot shower. Similarly, you can facilitate your hand and foot exercises with a sink or basin of warm water.

Active warm-ups for aerobic activity involve motion, but we don't want you to overdo it. The best way to warm up for walking, for example, is to start walking slowly. After about ten minutes, as your body heats up through increased blood circulation, you can pick up your pace with confidence. Elaborate stretches before walking may actually involve more muscle exertion—and danger of injury—than a series of slow, steady steps. Your regular arthritis exercise stretching and strengthening routine, however, would no doubt serve as excellent preparation for your aerobics, provided you have the *time* and *energy* to do everything in one fell swoop.

Cool-down after exercise is just as important as warm-up before. Slowing your pace as you come to the end of your aerobics is part of cooling down. So is a graceful flourish to your final stretch, accompanied by a few deep breaths. Many people like to relax with an ice pack for about ten minutes in the afterglow of a good workout. You will probably need at least ten minutes to return your heart rate to normal.

Motivational Strategy

No one knows better than you do what strategies will work to keep your motivation high. Are you a persevering sort who never waivers after making a decision? Or are you likely to lose interest in this new endeavor during the several weeks it may take to see real results? Are you a loner who will happily strike out for an early-morning walk before going to work? Or do you prefer a social setting for exercise—walking with a group of friends, say, or working out in a gym?

Taking stock of yourself now and planning what to do if and when you lose the urge to exercise can help you over the hard spots.

Here are some suggestions that may help keep you on track:

- Keep a log of your exercise progress, and the improvements in your condition.
- Set aside a place for your exercise, with everything you need handy—exercise equipment, mats, music, a special warm-up suit, etc.
- Arrange to exercise regularly with a friend or in a group, to put your exercise in a social context.
- Schedule a time of day that you can devote to exercise, and don't let anything else cut into that time. Exercise is *important.*
- Ask your doctor to help you compile a list of vital statistics, including weight, blood pressure, cholesterol level (including the percentage of high- and low-density lipoproteins), and sedimentation rate (for rheumatoid arthritis). After two months of regular exercise, take the profile again and see how the numbers have changed.
- Sit down and write yourself a letter, explaining your goals and hopes. Put it away somewhere. You may never need to look at it again, but if you find yourself looking for excuses to avoid exercise, take out the letter and read it.

CHAPTER 5

Relaxation Exercises

How to tap the energizing power of meditation

and other techniques that focus the mind

All physical exercises tend to benefit the mind as well as the body, by invigorating the spirits. The emphasis in this chapter, however, is on thought exercises that relax the mind and thereby relieve the body of the negative effects of stress.

Relaxation exercises require no physical exertion. They include deep breathing, progressive relaxation, imagery (visualization), and meditation. A time investment of as little as ten or twenty minutes a day spent in one of these quiet activities may result in a significant degree of pain reduction. What's more, these exercises can result in other positive physical effects, such as decreased blood pressure and heightened immunity to disease, as documented in medical studies.

Stress aggravates arthritis pain for 670 of our 1,051 Arthritis Survey participants—fully sixty-four percent of the survey group. It isn't that their ailments are caused by emotional problems, to be sure; it's just that stress can make arthritis symptoms flare. By the same token, the relief of stress may quiet those symptoms. For this reason, hundreds of our survey respondents relied on the relaxation exercises outlined here to get arthritis relief.

Deep breathing

Meditation and other formal relaxation techniques all begin by focusing the attention on breathing. This ploy takes your mind off external concerns and helps you gain active control over your body. When you breathe deeply you slow the rate of your breathing by taking a few big breaths instead of many small ones. Deep breathing often works quickly to block the more unpleasant aspects of stress, such as the painful pounding of a racing heart or tight muscles that are cramped with tension.

Inhale through your nose for several seconds, letting your chest expand fully. Try not to raise your shoulders as you inhale, as this motion does not help the lungs fill with air. Concentrate instead on widening the girth of your chest, picturing it inflating like a balloon. Your abdomen will expand, too, as your diaphragm drops down to increase the influx of air into the lungs.

Hold your breath for just a moment or two, and then slowly, slowly let it out through your mouth. As you exhale, picture your diaphragm rising and your chest contracting, as though squeezing the air out of your lungs. Picture physical tension leaving your body with each exhalation.

Once you become accustomed to deep breathing, and experiencing the comfort it brings, you may use it periodically throughout the day, any time something unpleasant jars you. Also try deep breathing as you go to sleep and again upon awakening.

Progressive Relaxation

This technique helps you achieve relaxed muscles by first reminding you how it feels to be all tensed up. The goal is to work and then relax all your muscles in order—starting from the face and proceeding down, or beginning at the feet, according to your preference.

Start by lying in a comfortable position with your eyes closed. Wriggle around a bit, then lie still and breathe deeply. If you are working with your feet first, tighten the toes and arches of one foot as hard as you can, hold briefly, and then let the muscles go limp. Do the same with the other foot.

Now tense one whole leg, straightening the knee and lifting the leg slightly to add to the tension. Then let the leg relax and slump back into place. Do the same with the other leg.

Continue on up your body, first tensing your abdomen and buttocks, then relaxing them completely. Clench each fist before you let your hands relax. Tense each arm and lift it and then let it fall limp at your side.

You can tense your neck by raising your head slightly, then lying back again. The muscles of your face can screw themselves into a sneer, fabricate an exaggerated grin, and knit your eyebrows to wrinkle your forehead.

When you have completed all these movements, lie still and concentrate on your breathing.

Imagery

Positive images, perhaps of beautiful places that you conjure up and elaborate upon in your mind, can have a powerfully soothing effect. Just as you can work yourself into a state of agitation by, for example, imagining an angry confrontation with your spouse, you can create the experience of deep relaxation by picturing a scene by some pleasant mountain stream, for example, smelling the grass and feeling the warm sunshine on your back as you watch the deer gather to drink there. Some people are able to use just such an imagined haven as a refuge from pain.

Many "guided imagery" tape recordings are available that can help you paint the details of pleasant scenes, in case you feel your own imagination isn't up to the task.

Meditation

With its long history in Eastern traditions, meditation has won new converts among medical doctors in recent decades because of its boon to health and well-being. Meditation brings on what Dr. Herbert Benson of Harvard Medical School has called "the relaxation response." This is a physiological state of deep rest. People experiencing the relaxation response are wide awake, but calm and refreshed. They may continue to feel the positive effects of twenty minutes' meditation throughout the day. You can, too.

Many books describe meditation techniques and practices. The basic outline here is drawn from one of Dr. Benson's books, called *Your Maximum Mind*.

- Begin by choosing a word or phrase that you can use as a focus for the meditation exercise. This could be a pleasant thought, such as "peace," or the opening of a prayer, or even a soothing sound that has no real meaning.
- Seat yourself in a comfortable position with your eyes closed and your muscles relaxed.
- As you breathe deeply, repeat your focus word or phrase to yourself with each exhalation.
- If worries or other thoughts come into your mind, calmly shoo them out again by repeating your focus word or phrase.
- Continue in this fashion for ten or twenty minutes.

These are the basic steps of meditation. Don't let the simplicity fool you into thinking that there's nothing much to it. Total concentration and the relaxation it brings will improve with practice, and may improve your quality of life significantly. If you want to make more of it, set aside a special place for meditation, where you keep a few favorite items that evoke positive feelings. Set aside a particular time of day, too, when you are least likely to be distracted. Ask your family and friends not to call you at this time. Take the telephone off the hook, or let the answering machine pick up, just to be safe.

We have considered each of these relaxation exercises separately, but they are easily combined. You may find, for example, that you can introduce a favorite image into your meditation, replacing your focus word or phrase with pictures. Deep breathing figures importantly in meditation, and also facilitates imagery.

Now that you are completely relaxed, you're ready to start your aerobic exercise.

P A R T
T H R E E

Aerobic Fitness Exercises for Arthritis

> Walking has a global effect on the entire person. It adds hours to one's day and years to one's life. Walking is a superior way to handle stress, and provides the isolation needed for meditation. Not the least of its benefits is the opportunity it gives for creative thinking and solving life's problems.
>
> If these rewards seem similar to the claims made by runners and cyclists and adherents of other activities, it is because they are. Exercise is the generic drug.
>
> —George Sheehan, M.D. from the preface to *Walking* by Casey Meyers

CHAPTER 6

Walking

How to turn an activity you've done all your life
into a safe, beneficial aerobic exercise

Walking is the oldest and best of the weight-bearing exercises for people with arthritis. We recommend it over jogging. More than half of the participants in our Arthritis Survey reported that they walk regularly for fitness and to maintain maximum mobility.

Jogging causes so many injuries that even young, athletic exercisers often choose to walk or swim instead. People with arthritis must be extra careful about any exercise that bounces and shocks the joints the way jogging does. And yet, some aerobic activity is crucial in the treatment of arthritis because it helps all the muscles and joints by increasing the blood flow to affected areas.

Luckily, numerous activities other than jogging can give the heart and lungs the necessary workout to improve circulation and stamina. Walking, generally considered the best aerobic exercise for people with arthritis, is easy, accessible, effective, and enjoyable. It can be geared to any level of fitness, and pursued by people of all ages.

Hospital studies show that walkers accrue the same cardiovascular benefits as runners, and with far fewer injuries. More to the point, clinical investigations document the fact that walking decreases arthritis pain. One hundred and two individuals with osteoarthritis recently participated in a study to test the benefits of walking, conducted at New York's Hospital for Special Surgery. The walkers in the group, who trekked for thirty minutes, three times a week for two months, experienced such significant levels of pain reduction that many were able to decrease the amount of medication they used.

Walking makes an ideal arthritis exercise because it is low-impact yet high-endurance once individuals build up to relatively long walks several times a week. Many formerly sedentary arthritis sufferers from our original survey group reported that they had transformed themselves into inveterate and hardy walkers. One woman, after many years spent in an extremely limited life-style, turned over a new, more active leaf by walking fifty feet a day.

A fitness exercise such as walking offers particular advantages to women because it can help prevent osteoporosis by strengthening the bones. Some researchers have found that exercise, coupled with calcium supplements, can even help prevent osteoporosis among women who are already past menopause.

No exercise could be more convenient than walking. You need no special equipment and no special clothing, other than comfortable shoes. You don't have to travel to the tennis court, the gym, the pool, or the golf course, you just get up and go. You can easily fit walking into your daily activities. Sometimes you can even fit your daily activities, such as shopping or doing errands, into your walk. And although walking will quicken your heart rate and get your body into condition, it won't make you perspire enough to require a shower or change of clothing immediately afterwards.

The number of times per week that you walk and the length of time you spend walking during each aerobic exercise session will depend on your level of exercise readiness. If you have been extremely limited in your activities because of pain or disability, your first goal may be to walk five minutes at a time in your own home, or around the block.

If you have fallen into inactivity by habit instead of being forced into it by pain, you may be able to start out by walking—slowly at first—for twenty minutes at a time, four times a week. Then you can increase the distance you walk, or the time you spend walking, or both, each week, until you are up to three or even four miles in an hour, five to seven days a week.

Remember, though, that persistence is more important than pace. No matter how slowly you walk, your joints will reap the benefits of exercise, and your heart will, too. A recent study at the famed Cooper Institute for Aerobics Research in Dallas demonstrated this surprising fact.* Dr. John Duncan recruited women who had been leading sedentary lives, and

---

*The Cooper Aerobics Center, founded by Ken Cooper in Dallas in the early 1970s, is comprised of the Cooper Clinic, a preventive and rehabilitative medicine facility; the Cooper Institute for Aerobics Research, where researchers study the role of exercise and other lifestyle factors in the maintenance of health; the Cooper Wellness Program, which provides a supportive, live-in environment where participants can focus time and attention on the challenging task of how to make positive lifestyle changes; and the Cooper Fitness Center, a health club in which all members' exercise efforts are supervised by a well-trained staff of health professionals.

put them on one of several walking programs. Once they got up to snuff, the three groups of walkers all showed up at the track five days a week and covered the same amount of ground, but in different periods of time: aerobic walkers finished the three-mile course in thirty-six minutes, brisk walkers took forty-six minutes, and slow strollers required a full hour to go the whole distance. Reporting his results in the *Journal of the American Medical Association,* Dr. Duncan said that although the aerobic walkers huffed and puffed the most and burned the most oxygen, all three groups showed the *same* healthful changes in their cholesterol levels.

Dr. James Rippe, director of the Exercise Physiology and Nutrition Laboratory at the University of Massachusetts School of Medicine, offers this sage advice to new walkers on how fast to step: "Walk as though you have someplace to go."

Dress for comfort and according to the weather. A good formula for cold weather is to dress in layers. These tend to hold in warmth, and you can always remove a layer or two if you feel too warm. In summer, even when you dress in light clothing, be alert for signs of heat stroke if you are a fast walker. The symptoms of this dangerous overheating include dizziness, headache, nausea, and cramping.

Give careful thought to the place you go for your walk. At first, select a round-trip route that you can complete in a reasonable amount of time. Later, as you walk more, you may want to change your destination. If you have a path or trail near you that promises the added bonus of beautiful scenery, so much the better.

Some people prefer to walk on grass or the soft surface of an artificially surfaced indoor track, as they feel it reduces the impact on the joints in their feet and ankles. Others find they can manage well on a sidewalk, so long as their walking shoes provide good cushioning.

Once you get out and about, you will notice the exercise habits of other walkers, many of whom dress in elegant sweat suits and fancy walking shoes. You'll see that some of them walk with one finger pressed against the side of the neck, or the opposite wrist, to check their pulse and make sure they've got their hearts pumping at the ideal rate. A few very serious walkers may even sport sophisticated wrist meters, with enough tiny dials to satisfy a jet pilot, on which they monitor their vital functions. You can take the exercise as far as you like for maximum fitness, but the primary goal in arthritis care is simply to keep your body moving and bearing its own weight.

If you have an uneven gait, or walk with a limp, make sure that walking for aerobic exercise does not exacerbate your condition. Try to walk at a slow pace, taking smaller than usual steps, if necessary, so that you maintain as even a stride as possible. Otherwise, you may place undue strain on several joints. When walking with a cane, hold it in the hand opposite the affected leg. (If it's your right hip or ankle that pains you, hold the cane in your left hand.)

Breathe deeply and evenly as you walk, and swing or pump your arms. Also, try to maintain your best posture, looking straight ahead of you, with your head up, chest out, shoulders back but relaxed, hips tucked under, and tummy in.

As for time spent walking, any amount of time is better than no time. According to an earlier, larger study at the Cooper Clinic, headed by Dr. Steven N. Blair, walking as little as half an hour a day can increase a person's longevity by warding off two of the leading killers—heart disease and cancer.

Walking works wonders. But how can you make yourself undertake the work of walking? Try walking one or more of the following ways:

- Around the track at your local high school
- On a beach or through the woods where beauty surrounds you
- On a treadmill while reading the newspaper or watching the television news

- Along a sidewalk looking at the passersby and the store window displays
- Through a shopping mall in any weather
- With a friend or family member
- With your pet
- To and from work
- On your errands
- Listening to music on a portable radio
- Listening to taped lectures or talking books on a small tape player with headphones
- Letting your mind run free to dream up creative ideas
- Even on days that aren't balmy, sunny, and bright
- At dawn, to start the day off right
- During lunch hour, as a break from the day's other activities
- In the evening, when the full moon can be your night light

Because walking came naturally to you in childhood, you may take it for granted now. All the fuss made over it in books and magazines may seem misplaced, but keeping the activity's advantages in mind can help you adhere to your exercise regimen. Remember, brisk walking gives you a good workout that will benefit your heart as much as your joints. What's more, since most people can walk for a longer time than they could run or play tennis, walking tends to build muscular endurance while it burns calories. And walking is so accessible and easy to do that you're far less likely to quit this exercise regimen than any other you might try.

CHAPTER 7

Swimming and Water Exercises

How to find your way to healthy workouts

in the water—even if you can't swim a stroke

Water's buoyancy makes swimming virtually a no-impact aerobic activity. If you don't know how to swim, you can learn now, taking advantage of the many courses offered at health clubs, YMCAs/YMHAs, and schools. If you don't care to take the plunge, remember that being a nonswimmer need not stop you from venturing into the shallow end of a warm pool and doing your range-of-motion exercises there, or splashing around to give your joints a good workout. You may also find that just being in the water relaxes you and further reduces your pain, especially if it's in the comfortable range of 86 degrees Fahrenheit.

Even jogging becomes a safe, sane exercise for people with arthritis when they jog in waist-deep water! It's well-nigh impossible to sustain an impact injury while jogging in a swimming pool. Your bones don't take a pounding when you water-jog, even when you vary your pace from a slow gait to a faster one. The deeper you submerge yourself in the water, the less you stress your joints as you jog or walk. Try these activities first in waist-level water, then in water up to your shoulders to see the difference for yourself. You can also run in the deep water, where your feet will never touch the bottom of the pool, but your arms and legs will have to pump and cycle, respectively, to propel you forward. You'll be in good company: remember that superstar runners including Mary Decker Slaney maintain fitness while recovering from injuries by running in water.

Swimming counts as an ideal aerobic exercise because it makes both the arms and the legs work hard, and gets the heart pumping.

Some experts, however, argue that swimming is no match for walking or running as a weight-bearing exercise. While it's true that the water provides a virtually stress-free environment for the bones and joints, swimmers have been shown to have thicker, stronger bones than people who perform no exercise.

Perhaps you used to be a good swimmer, but arthritis has cramped your style, making it hard for you to turn your head in proper form for breathing while swimming the crawl. Try using a snorkel—the kind skindivers wear—so you can breathe easily without overexerting your neck muscles. Even though this technique has been used with great success in hospital studies, some people find that the sidestroke, with its more gentle action, works better for them than the crawl. You can experiment with different strokes until you find the one that suits you best. You can also combine a variety of strokes to add interest to your swimming. By alternating between difficult and simple strokes, you can pace yourself, getting a good workout while avoiding rapid fatigue.

If your legs are in great shape but your arms or shoulders are too weak to swim yet, you can still start out in the pool by using a kickboard. This aid allows you to kick to your heart's content and propel yourself across the pool while your arms do hardly any work at all.

Warm up for swimming by performing a few range-of-motion exercises at the side of the pool before you break into your laps.

More than 200 of our original Arthritis Survey respondents made the effort to get to a pool regularly, even if it meant traveling by bus at considerable inconvenience. The return on their time investment paid off in terms of decreased pain, they reported. Those who had to pay for pool time by joining a health club reasoned that they were saving money in the long run—by cutting their monthly costs for pain medications.

We encourage you to try out the pool at the club before you join. If the water is too cold, or if there are too many people swimming laps at the hours you hope to exercise, you will not be able to fulfill your needs. More than likely, you'll have several pool facilities to choose from, and can find one that suits you perfectly.

Another advantage of water is that it makes exercise a virtually no-sweat proposition. The reason is that water is much more efficient than air at dissipating heat—four times as efficient, to be exact. The result is that your body doesn't get overheated and you can continue to feel comfortable even though you're working hard in hot weather.

If you perform your stretching and strengthening exercises in a pool, you'll find that the water gives just enough resistance to add an extra degree of muscle building to many of these maneuvers. Some movements, on the other hand, actually become easier. For example, you'll find that a standing knee-to-chest stretch or a straight leg-up raise can be performed with reduced effort when your legs are buoyed by water.

When you first begin aquatic exercise, or whenever you need a little added support, you can wear a buoyancy vest or belt to help you stay upright as you work out in the water.

At the pool, as on the walking paths, you'll encounter the advanced equipment of enthusiasts, such as water dumbbells and weighted benches for transferring bench or step aerobics to the water setting. The SelfCare Catalog, a popular mail order source for health care products, offers a full page of water-fitness gear. Items include a "Swim-in-Place Stretch Cord" for people with lots of determination but little room to swim in, that lets you tether yourself to your pool's ladder and swim as long as you like without going anywhere; a water-proof ring that will keep track of the number of laps you swim; a buoyancy belt; water dumbbells; zero-impact footwear that purports to help you gain added strength in your legs from deep-water running; and high-top water shoes that can be worn in the pool or out. (For more information on any of these products, call the company's order line at 1–800–345–3371.) Depending on your level of ability (and income!), you may want to try some of these exercise aids, but the water itself suffices for most people.

Given the popularity of exercise and the increased availability of swimming pools, more and more people are pursuing aquatic aerobics. The American Fitness Association in Durango, Colorado, estimates that the number of individuals getting fit in the water has increased from about 500,000 in 1986 to more than four and a half million in 1992. Many of these individuals have arthritis.

CHAPTER 8

Cycling

How to use bicycles, indoors or out, in a low-impact aerobic exercise program for arthritis

Cycling is a good aerobic activity for people with arthritis because it involves an even lower level of impact than walking. We're talking about the normal leg motion here, of course. If you fall off the bicycle, the impact is stunning!

Cycling enthusiasts say that this sport is so gentle on the body it can even be pursued by people who can't walk. Some doctors, however, counter that cycling is great for the hips, but not so great for the knees. From what we can determine, some knee problems attributed to cycling are really due to riding bikes with pedals set at improper heights, or to overexertion in cycling that pushes the legs too far, too fast, before muscles adapt to the exercise. Do exercise with caution: cycling may aggravate *your* knees.

Numerous clinical studies have demonstrated the benefits of bicycling in the overall treatment of arthritis. One study involved twenty-three women with rheumatoid arthritis who exercised with stationary bicycles, but at different levels of difficulty and for varying periods of time. Even those women who exercised for just fifteen minutes per session found that they developed greater strength and endurance, and that fewer of their joints felt painful and swollen. In another study, the subjects who rode stationary bicycles achieved the same overall flexibility as another group who did only flexibility (range-of-motion) exercises—and increased their endurance as well. In yet another study that included cycling as part of an exercise regimen, most of the subjects felt so much improved by the time the research program ended that they continued to follow the routine on their own.

Equipment becomes an important consideration in cycling, as bicycles with many gears offer the most options to people with arthritis. Riding a bike gets you out and about, making it an appealing pastime. Do be sure to pay close attention to safety, however. Now that the pattern of injuries incurred while bicycling is well-known, every cyclist needs to wear a helmet. Even top pros who have never fallen off a bike in their lives avow that head protection is essential, whether riding on special bicycle paths or on streets shared with auto traffic. Night riders need reflectors on the bicycle itself, as well as on their clothing and helmet. It's also a good idea to equip your bicycle with head- and taillights.

The racing bike, which requires the rider to assume a near-fetal position and then crane his neck up to see straight ahead, has at last given way in popularity to the upright touring and all-terrain bikes. This trend is a real boon to people with arthritis. You will be much more comfortable sitting straight up than hunching over for the sake of reducing air resistance on your body. When you are riding to gain exercise and fresh air, as opposed to winning first place in the *Tour de France*,* sitting up is the position of choice.

A bicycle has to fit its rider for comfort and efficiency. This is generally true, but especially important for people with arthritis, to avoid added stress on any joint. A reputable bicycle dealer will ask you to sit on the bike before you buy it, and then adjust the seat so that you can almost but not quite straighten your leg when you have pushed the pedal as far down as it will go. Also, you need an optimal distance between the seat and the handlebars, or you will develop back pain from overreaching. This distance is defined by the length of the rider's forearm, from the elbow to the tips of the fingers. (Sometimes the handlebar distance looks right on purchase, but will need adjusting later, either by tilting the seat or changing the bars so that they extend farther back.)

The gears on the bicycle function to give you an energy advantage. Used properly, they improve your pedaling efficiency, so that you can keep up the same rate of leg work whether you're on a hill or a level surface. They have nothing to do with speed, so you need not be scared away from a ten-or-more-speed bicycle just because you're not planning to go very fast. A "ten-speed" bicycle should really be called a "ten-gear" bicycle. After all, no bicycle can go faster than you can pedal it, no matter how many gears it has.

Most adult bikes come equipped with hand brakes. If you have the hand strength to operate these brakes, do check to see that your hands can comfortably span the distance (called the "reach") between the handlebars and brake levers. If you have trouble using your hands, you may want to try to find a bicycle with foot brakes instead.

*The *Tour de France* is a three-week bicycle race that covers more than 2,000 miles.

When you ride, put the balls of your feet on the pedals.

Cycling can now be enjoyed as an indoor as well as an outdoor sport. Exercycles rooted to one spot in your home can be adjusted to offer minimal resistance when easy riding is required. You can reduce the tension to zero, if need be, or raise it to mimic the steepest hillside imaginable. These indoor bicycles go by many names, such as "stationary cycle," for obvious reasons, and "bicycle ergometer," which is the term physical therapists prefer, because it emphasizes the point that you can measure the amount of work you're doing as you spin your wheels. (The hospital studies mentioned above were all performed with bicycle ergometers.)

We think of cycling as legwork, and it is, but some stationary cycles include activities for the arms as well. As you pump the pedals with your feet, you grasp handles that you push/pull back and forth with your arms. There are even cycle ergometers designed expressly for upper-body work, and these offer an alternative to people whose legs can't take the strain of most aerobic activities.

Seat comfort is an all-important consideration. Whether you ride indoors or out, you need to remain seated throughout your workout. Some people will experience nothing more annoying than a mild soreness the first few days of getting used to a bicycle seat. Others find the pain in their buttocks never goes away. If you are in this latter category, cycling is not for you. Before you give up the advantages of the sport, however, try to make your bike seat as comfortable as you can with a padded seat cover, or even by changing the seat (to one often called a saddle) altogether until you find one that you can tolerate.

Add another level of comfort to your riding by wearing padded gloves. These bicycle gloves, which are perforated for use in warm weather, were originally introduced to give serious racers a better grip and greater comfort during long rides. If you don't like them or find them too expensive, then by all means build up the grips on your handle bars with foam padding. You can purchase large, soft grips at bicycle stores, or you can make your own out of layers of foam.

Stationary cycling combines itself easily with other activities. Many people find their exercise period the ideal time to read a book or magazine, watch the news on television, or see a movie on the VCR.

CHAPTER 9

Dancing and More

How to set your aerobic workout to music

and step through it with rhythm and pleasure

The best exercise regimens are often the ones that provide a real recreational and social outlet, so that they not only improve your physical condition but put you in the swing of things and make you feel good to be alive.

Dancing provides this combination of good movements and good times with others. Ballroom dancing in particular, with its built-in opportunities to rest between numbers, is becoming a favorite exercise pastime. Folk dancing, even more than couples dancing, brings groups of people together for active recreation. There are even a few specialized dance schools that cater to people with arthritis.

At least one hospital study has shown that the rigors of aerobic dance, believe it or not, can be modified to make this popular activity low-impact enough for people with arthritis —and beneficial for them, too.

Dancing combines range-of-motion maneuvers and strengthening exercises in the prescribed steps. When you dance to the music of a song set, continuing until the music ends, you get built-in repetitions of the movements, not to mention endurance training. What's more, dancing definitely drives depression away with its strong positive effect on the spirits. The chance to be with other people in an active form of recreation makes dancing virtually boredom-proof. People may abandon their exercycles and find excuses to avoid the swimming pool on a chilly day, but dancing retains its appeal over the long haul. It's really a fun way to rediscover how much your body can do.

Health experts consider dancing a reasonable alternative to other aerobic activities, including walking, swimming, cycling, and jogging.

"Ya gotta keep dancing!" several of our Arthritis Survey participants maintained.

One of the chief benefits of dancing is the relaxed style of movement that comes from mastering steps to music. As dancers become accustomed to rhythmically positioning their bodies in space, they find that they develop dancelike ways of doing other activities. Their motions may become more fluid, so that they stop walking with a stiff-legged gait. Instead of striking rigid poses while they stand at the kitchen counter or sit at a desk, for example, they bring the good body mechanics of dancing to bear by adding a little motion. Some dancers gently dip and shift their weight from one leg to the other while working standing up, or perform a rock-and-roll stretch of the lower back while typing at the computer keyboard.

If you've never danced before, you'll want to do some at-home preparation before you take to the dance floor. Your regular range-of-motion and strengthening exercises, outlined in part 4, will get your body ready for new moves. If you're worried about catching your breath while you're keeping step to the beat, remember that you can gain an aerobic advantage by starting to walk regularly.

In discussing your exercise plans with your doctor, check to see if there's any reason that dancing might cause a problem for you. Even if you have artificial joints in your hips or knees, or a tendency to accumulate fluid in these joints, you will more than likely be able to hit on safe ways to approach the dance floor.

The best way to determine the best type of dancing for you is by assessing your joint condition. Painful hands are best held gently by a ballroom partner—not allemanded left and right in a square dance setting where you can't control who will grasp your hand, or how vigorously. However, your toes will less likely get stepped on while folk dancing, where partners tend to hold each other at arm's length. You can keep an even greater distance from your fellow dancers by taking a class in modern dance or jazzercise. That way, you'll do the steps on your own, but you'll still be in a group of dancers where movement and music can improve your muscle tone and lift your spirits.

Ballet, especially in toe shoes, is generally considered too stressful for joints already stressed by arthritis. If, however, you can find a beginner's class with an understanding teacher, you may well find the disciplined, graceful exercises at the barre to be just what you need to improve your posture, muscle strength, and flexibility.

Should you decide to take formal lessons in social dancing, or dance/exercise classes, try to arrange a brief meeting with your instructor before classes begin, when you can talk candidly about your arthritis and any special concerns you might have. This gives you a chance to explain in advance that you may, for example, want to rest frequently at the outset, or avoid altogether any movements that seem to you to be too jarring. If you feel embarrassed about initiating such a discussion, you can always drop a note, but do let the instructor know what to expect from you in class.

Since you'll be on your feet and using them a great deal, you'll need supportive, comfortable dancing shoes. These can be of almost any variety, but low-heeled styles make the most sense. Classic saddle shoes, which were popular in the 1960s, are making a comeback these days—cushioning many dancing feet moving to the big band sound at swing-dance fests. The shoes fit right in with the period outfits that include full circle skirts and skinny ties. Their fit on the feet can be quite comfortable, too, given their good support, laces, and wide-toe box. Sturdy leather saddle shoes provide more protection from your partner's feet than any sneakers made of leather or canvas can!

Other Dancelike Disciplines

Some of the routinized movements from Oriental martial arts, such as karate and t'ai chi ch'uan, share the benefits of dance as a form of aerobic exercise. Karate, for one, includes stretching, isometric and isotonic strengthening, and aerobic activity. Just as dance combines these movement basics in a structure set to music, karate incorporates the elements of exercise in a technique with a long historic tradition and a philosophy of peace and harmony. Teachers of karate frequently speak of the discipline's emphasis on self-expression, and the way karate respects the needs and capabilities of each individual.

Movies have convinced many of us that karate is all about violence, or defending oneself against violence, but you can learn karate even if you have considerable physical limitation. More importantly, you can find arthritis relief in its movements.

CHAPTER 10

Exercise by Any Other Name

How to turn your chores and favorite pastimes into aerobic exercises that help keep you going strong

Everybody knows somebody who seems to be in great shape but swears that exercise is not the reason. These people can't be coaxed out for a walk, hate the idea of swimming laps, and equate exercycles with instruments of torture. Yet they carry themselves well, and can charge up the stairs without pausing to catch their breath. What's their secret?

They *are* exercising; they just don't know it. They pursue jobs, chores, or hobbies that confer all the advantages of aerobic exercise. They've been fooled into fitness by doing the things they have to do or the things they love to do.

In our original Arthritis Survey group, for example, were waitresses who spent hours on their feet, trekking back and forth to some restaurant's kitchen, carrying trayloads of dishes. This activity, though it cannot boast the relaxation of walking in the woods, certainly gets the heart pumping and the muscles contracting.

Other survey group participants, however, physically exerted themselves in pursuit of a favorite pastime. These individuals enjoyed a workout *and* a wonderful time.

Gardening exemplifies the kind of activity that combines aerobic, stretching, and strengthening exercises with the pursuit of pleasure. Gardening has shown itself to be the aerobic equal of walking for those people addicted to digging and planting. The excitement of tending the growing shoots makes the activity so engrossing that there is no problem in building up to a fitness level of endurance. On the contrary, gardeners with arthritis must often be dragged indoors against their will before they overexert themselves. It is not unusual to find someone forgetting all about pain during a two- or three-hour stint of hoeing and weeding in the garden.

If this sounds like your kind of exercise, try to keep the fitness goals in mind as you plan your vegetable or flower garden. Each time you go outdoors to do your gardening, try to vary the activities as much as possible. If you spend your whole time crouched down between the rows, for example, you not only miss out on aerobic exercise, but you will no doubt exacerbate stiffness in your legs. If weeding is the order of the day, try pulling weeds for twenty minutes, and then getting up to carry each small load to a compost heap or other disposal site.

Aim to maintain an awareness of your posture and movements as you work. This means keeping your back straight and bending with your knees when you must get down to ground level. Stay loose by occasionally shrugging and rolling your shoulders as you work. Carry flats or potted plants high and close to your body, so they don't force you to stoop over. For really heavy loads, use a wheelbarrow.

Equip yourself with any gardening tools that are specifically designed to make the job easier on your body. Some examples include:

- A soft pad to sit or kneel on while weeding
- A low stool as another comfort aid for weeding work
- A hose caddy
- Extra long–handled shovels, hoes, and rakes that enable you to stand up straight while working in the garden.

If you don't have a green thumb or any hope of developing one, you may find other aerobic-type physical outlets in and around your house. Yard work such as raking leaves qualifies. So do many aspects of home upkeep, including indoor and outdoor painting, polishing and refinishing old furniture finds, and giving your house a truly thorough cleaning. Laundry is another task that can be turned to aerobic advantage by ignoring a few modern conveniences and taking the wash outside to dry it on a clothesline.

Caring for and playing with young children—your own or someone else's—can give you an exhausting physical workout and much pleasure, too. Some people with arthritis fear that children will be too rough on them, or insist on playing active games that could tire out a young adult with no disabilities of any kind. However, even very young children can be taught to recognize and respect a caregiver's physical limitations. As long as they know they are getting an adult's full and willing attention, they are usually content to structure the play at the older person's pace.

Sexual activity also offers many of the same benefits as exercise, such as flooding the brain with endorphins that lift the spirits and quell pain. Sexual arousal also induces the body to release adrenalin and cortisone into the blood. These substances act as natural painkillers.

You may need to experiment with your partner to find the most comfortable positions for intercourse or other sex play. It goes without saying that aerobic activity will be the natural outcome of your enjoyment—not the primary goal!

As gerontologist Alex Comfort has remarked, "Most people can and should have sex long after they no longer wish to ride bicycles."

P A R T
F O U R

Exercising Away Pain from Head to Toe

> *Stretching, because it relaxes your mind and tunes up your body, should be part of your daily life.*
>
> —Bob Anderson
> author, *Stretching*

CHAPTER 11

Neck and Jaw Exercises

Specific exercises for two prime locations

of muscle tension and stress in the body

You can do your neck a lot of good by remembering that good posture starts at the head. As you go through the day, try to keep your head up and well aligned with the rest of your body. If you "lead with your chin" as you walk or work, you'll be scrunching together the seven vertebrae in your neck. Instead, keep your chin tucked in, just as you tuck in your tummy to straighten your back.

Move your neck as much as you can to keep its muscles relaxed. Many of us have a tendency to apply stress and tension directly to our neck muscles, holding them rigidly and aggravating pain in the neck!

The Yes-No and Left-Right exercises described on page 72 can be done anytime, anywhere, to loosen up a tight neck, as can parts of the Head Roll. Stress and tension may also express themselves in the jaw, through rigidly held "tight-lipped" expressions and grinding or clenching of the teeth.

The first exercise in the following group stretches the jaw, while the rest concentrate on the neck. They are arranged according to starting position, so that the first few can be done as part of an in-bed routine upon awakening.

If you have rheumatoid arthritis, please approach these exercises with caution, as the disease can make the neck joints extremely unstable. You'll want to stretch and strengthen your neck muscles gently and wisely. The advice, "Don't push beyond pain," is especially relevant here.

A-E-I-O-U SHOUT

Type: Stretching

Starting position: This exercise can be done in virtually any position.

Steps:
1. Pronounce or mouth the vowel sound "A" for several seconds, exaggerating the motion of your lips and jaw for maximum stretch. Your mouth should be wide open, as though you were cheering silently.
2. Say "E," drawing out the sound and baring your teeth like an angry cat.
3. Drop your jaw as far as possible to say "I" with the stretch of a big yawn.
4. Sustain the "O" sound, with rounded lips and raised eyebrows.
5. Push your lips far forward as you say "U" with "oomph."

SHOULDER SHRUG

Type: Stretching

Starting position: You can do this exercise lying in bed, sitting, or standing, with your arms at your sides.

Steps:
1. Slowly and steadily raise your shoulders to a shrug.
2. Hold for a moment, feeling the effect on your neck muscles.
3. Keeping your head still, gently press your shoulders as far down as you can.
4. Hold, feeling the stretch in your neck.

Note: This exercise benefits the shoulders and appears in that section as well.

BED HEAD

Type: Stretching and strengthening

Starting position: Lie on your back in bed or on the floor.

Steps:
1. Press your head straight back into your pillow or mat.
2. Hold for a moment, then release the pressure.
3. Lift your head above your pillow or mat as high as you can, without lifting your shoulders.
4. Hold, feeling the stretch in your neck, then release.

Note: Later in the day, you can repeat steps 1 and 2 of this exercise by pressing your head against your arm or a wall.

HEAD ROLL

Type: Stretching

Starting position: Sit in a chair or stand with your feet at a comfortable distance apart. Hold your head high and look straight ahead.

Steps:

1. Tilt your head to the left as though you were trying to put your ear on your shoulder. *a*

2. Stop when you've stretched your neck as far as you can. Don't try to bring your shoulder up to meet your ear.

3. Roll your head forward and down, as though trying to touch your chin to your chest. *b*

4. Continue the roll toward the right, as though trying to place your right ear on your right shoulder. *c*

5. Come full circle by tilting your head back, but not too far. *d*

6. Return to starting position.

7. Repeat these steps, circling your head to the right this time.

Note: If you have been advised not to tilt your head back, simply omit Step 5 of this exercise.

This exercise can be done in bed by modifying it slightly to omit the forward and backward motions. Simply slide and tilt your head to the left, then back up to the center, then to the right and back to center.

HEAD ROLL

Tilt your head to one side, then forward, then to the other side in a slow, continuous roll that gently stretches your neck muscles.

Try to move only your head and neck, keeping your shoulders level. (In other words, resist the temptation to raise your shoulder to your ear!)

The full circle includes a tilt back, too, but this part of the stretch is a problem for some people. If your neck hurts in this position, or if you have rheumatoid arthritis, leave out this step.

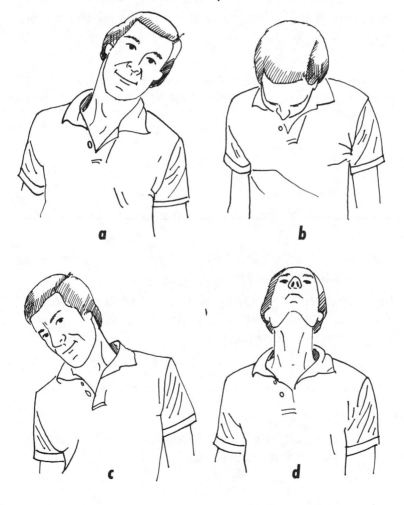

a

b

c

d

LEFT-RIGHT

Type: Stretching

Starting position: You can do this exercise lying in bed, sitting, or standing, with your arms at your sides.

Steps:
1. Keeping your head level, turn to the right as though trying to see behind your back.
2. Return your head and your gaze to center.
3. Turn your head to look toward the left as far as you can.
4. Return to starting position.

Advanced variation: After you have turned your head as far as possible, tilt it down as though trying to touch your chin to your shoulder.

YES-NO

Type: Stretching

Starting position: You may sit or stand virtually anywhere.

Steps:
1. Nod your head yes, slowly, several times. Keep your neck still but relaxed, moving only your head.
2. Turn your head side-to-side, as though making an exaggerated "no" gesture. Again, keep your neck still and move only your head.

HEAD PULL

Type: Stretching

Starting position: Sit in a chair with your back straight and your hands clasped behind your head.

Steps:

1. Gently pull your head forward and down to stretch the back of your neck.

2. Hold for a moment.

3. Return to your starting position.

NECK PUSH

Type: Strenghthening

Starting position: Sit or stand comfortably.

Steps:

1. Press the palm of one hand against your forehead, and your forehead against the palm of your hand.

2. Hold for a moment, keeping the pressure on your hand and head without moving either one.

3. Repeat with the other hand.

Note: If your hands and wrists are particularly painful, you may apply the pressure with your forearm. Another possibility is to press your head against a wall.

CHAPTER 12

Shoulder Exercises

How to shrug, roll, stretch, and strengthen the joints that carry the weight of the world

You really do carry the weight of the world on these body parts, lifting them (and consequently tensing your neck) to shoulder life's stresses and strains.

Your shoulders bear the distinction of being the most flexible joints in your body, when they are functioning smoothly. Since they are capable of so many kinds of motion, your exercise regimen will combine several movements to work your shoulders to their full potential.

Most shoulder exercises can be done one shoulder at a time, or both together, whichever way suits you better. Many of them also exercise the neck, arms, and hands.

If you use a cane to assist you while walking, you'll find that it makes an excellent baton for shoulder stretches. A few other simple aids to exercise that you may already have around the house include a clothesline for shoulder stretches and a couple of rice cartons or canned goods to be used as one-pound weights.

The most difficult shoulder exercises are those that ask you to extend your arms out straight at shoulder level, as in the Semaphore and the Crisscross.

SHOULDER SHRUG

Type: Stretching

Starting position: You can do this exercise lying in bed, sitting, or standing, with your arms at your sides.

Steps:
1. Slowly and steadily raise your shoulders to a shrug.
2. Hold for a moment, feeling the effect on your neck muscles.
3. Keeping your head still, gently press your shoulders as far down as you can.

Note: This exercise benefits the neck and appears in that section as well.

SWINGING PENDULUM

Type: Gentle stretching

Starting Position: In bed, lie face down near the edge of your bed, with one arm hanging free over the edge. (You'll need to roll to the opposite edge to repeat the exercise with your other shoulder.)

In a sitting or standing position, lean forward and let one or both arms hang down, straight but relaxed. You may work the shoulders individually or together.

Steps:

1. Swing your arm(s) gently to and fro, parallel to your body.
2. Swing your arm(s) gently out and back, perpendicular to your body.
3. Swing your arm(s) in small circles, first to the left, then to the right.

SHOULDER HELPER

Type: Very gentle range-of-motion exercise

Starting position: Sit in a chair.

Steps:

1. Put your right hand on your left shoulder and gently lift the shoulder as far as it will go.
2. Still using your right hand, press the left shoulder down as far as you can.
3. Pull your shoulder forward to its limit.
4. Push your shoulder back as far as possible.
5. Using your left hand on your right shoulder, repeat the above steps.

SHOULDER ROLL

Type: Stretching

Starting position: You may sit or stand with your shoulders relaxed. Try to proceed through the steps in one fluid motion, making a circle with your shoulder(s).

Steps:

1. Raise your shoulder(s).
2. Bring your shoulder(s) forward.

SHOULDER ROLL, continued

3. Push your shoulder(s) down.
4. Pull your shoulder(s) back.
5. Return to starting position.
6. Circle your shoulder(s) in the opposite direction (reversing the order of Steps 1–4).

WALL WALKER

Type: Stretching

Starting position: You may stand or sit about two feet away from a wall, with your left side to the wall, arms at your sides.

Steps:
1. Let your left hand slowly "walk" up the wall, as though your fingers were the legs of an insect. *a*
2. "Walk" above shoulder level if you can, but try not to raise your shoulder or lean away from the wall. "Let your fingers do the walking." *b*
3. Turn and "walk" your right hand.

Note: This exercise is also included in the Hands/Fingers section, as it benefits those joints as well.

BUTTERFLY STRETCH

Type: Stretching

Starting position: Sit in a chair or stand at ease, arms at your sides.

Steps:
1. Clasp your hands behind your head.
2. Open your elbows out to your sides as far as you can.

3. Bring your elbows together in front of you, making them meet, if possible.

4. Return to starting position.

5. Place your fingertips on your shoulders, elbows pointing out to the sides.

6. Pull your elbows back as far as you can.

7. Push your elbows forward and try to touch them together.

8. Return to starting position.

SEMAPHORE

Type: Stretching

Starting position: You may sit in a straight-back chair or stand at ease, arms at your sides.

Steps:

1. Extend your arms straight out to the sides at shoulder height. *a*

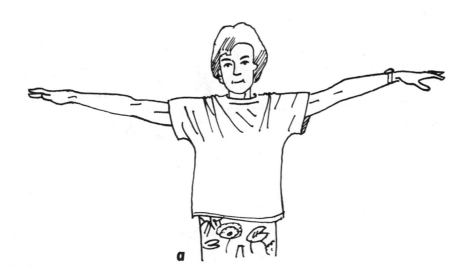

a

SEMAPHORE, continued

2. Keeping your arms straight and at shoulder height, touch your hands together in front. **b**

3. Move your arms back out to your sides. **c**

4. Still keeping your arms at shoulder height, move them as though you could touch your hands together in back. **d**

5. Extend your arms out to the sides again. **e**

6. Raise both arms straight up, biceps close to your ears. **f**

7. Lower your arms and let them hang at your sides.

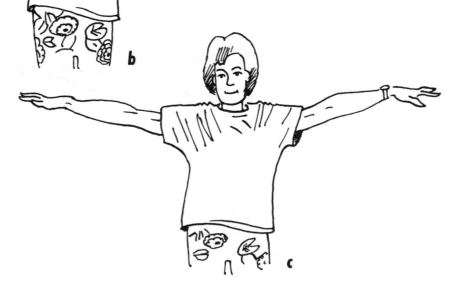

SEMAPHORE

If you put a couple of signal flags in your hands, these stretching motions might well send important messages!

Remember to keep your elbows straight and your arms at shoulder height as you do your flag-waving.

b

c

Note: *Figure d is shown from a different perspective to show the full stretch from behind. You are not expected to change positions.*

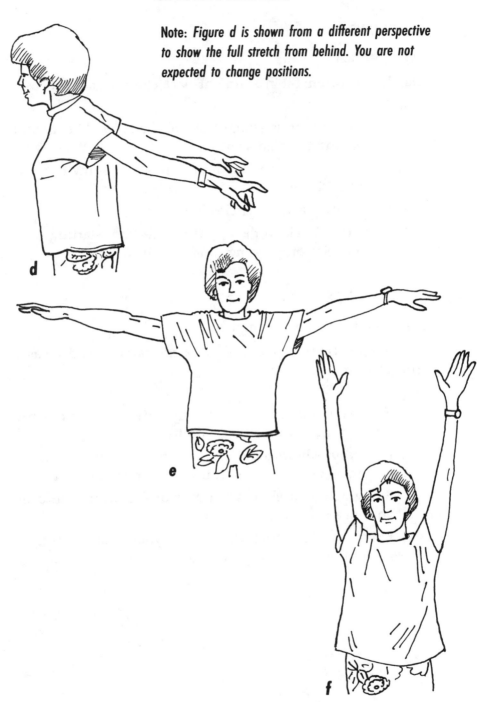

d

e

f

81

CIRCLING

Type: Stretching

Starting position: Sit in a straight-back chair or stand at ease.

Steps:
1. Extend your arms straight out to the sides, like a child pretending to be an airplane.
2. Move your arms so that your hands make tiny forward circles in the air.
3. Gradually make the circles larger.
4. Stop, then circle in the opposite direction, starting with small circles progressing to larger ones.

BODYBUILDER

Type: Stretching and strengthening

Starting position: Sit in a straight-back chair or stand at ease, arms at your sides.

Steps:
1. Raise your arms straight out to the sides with your palms up, and make your hands into fists.
2. Bend your elbows to bring your fists over your shoulders, raising as big a bulge as you can in your biceps. *a*
3. Straighten your elbows to put your fists in the air, over your head. *b*
4. Bring your fists back down over your shoulders, then straight out, then drop them down at your sides.

BODYBUILDER

Whether or not you raise big bulges in your biceps as you go through these motions, you'll stretch and strengthen the muscles of your upper arms and shoulders.

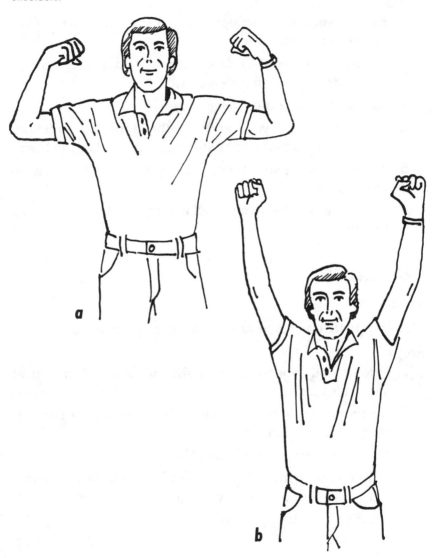

CIRCLE TWIST

Type: Stretching

Starting position: Sit in a straight-back chair or stand at ease.

Steps:

1. Extend your arms straight out to the sides, with your palms facing the floor.
2. Clench your hands in fists and move your arms so that your fists make tiny forward circles.
3. Gradually make the circles larger.
4. Stop and rotate your arms in the opposite direction, starting with small circles and gradually enlarging them.
5. Twist your arms so that your palms (still clenched in fists) face the ceiling.
6. Now make circles, from small to large, first forward, then backward.

CRISSCROSS

Type: Stretching

Starting position: Stand at ease, arms at your sides.

Steps:

1. Extend both your arms straight out in front of you at shoulder height.
2. Keeping arms straight, cross the right one over the left, then left over right. *a*
3. Move your arms out to the sides.
4. Lower your arms and try to cross your wrists in back, right over left, and left over right. *b*
5. Return to starting position.

CRISSCROSS

With your arms in front, you may well be able to cross them at the elbows and perform a scissors-like motion the first time you try this exercise.

When you reach behind yourself, you'll find you get enough of a stretch by crossing your arms at your wrists.

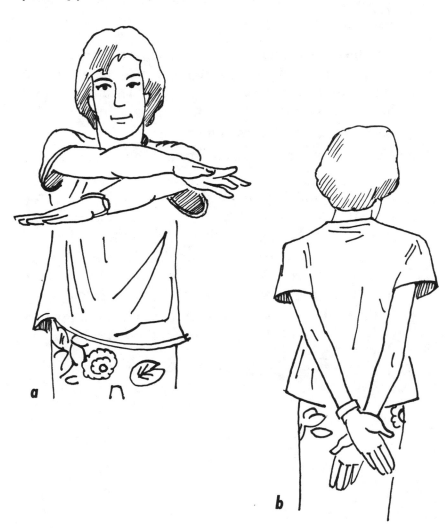

a

b

STRAIGHT EDGE

Type: Stretching

Starting position: You may sit in a chair or stand at ease. You will need a cane (or a yardstick, broom handle, or exercise baton). Have your arms hanging relaxed, one end of the cane in each hand.

Steps:

1. Lift the cane as high over your head as possible. (If you have more mobility in one shoulder than the other, then your cane will make a diagonal line, instead of a horizontal line, above you.) *a*

2. Lower the cane and rest a moment.

3. Hold the cane straight out in front of you, about shoulder height.

4. Using both arms, move the cane to the right and then to the left. Try to keep your back and hips still as you do this, concentrating on moving your shoulders. *b*

5. Holding the cane out front at shoulder level, and keeping both hands on it, lift and lower first one end of the cane, then the other. (Rest here again, if you need to.) *c*

6. Lift the cane over your head and then bring it down to shoulder height behind your head. (You may bend your head forward.) *d*

7. Return to starting position.

STRAIGHT EDGE

Try to keep your cane at shoulder height for maximum benefit as you go through these motions. (You may need to start at a lower height than shown in the illustration.)

If one of your shoulders is more restricted than the other, then just raise that arm as high as you comfortably can, and don't worry if your cane slants.

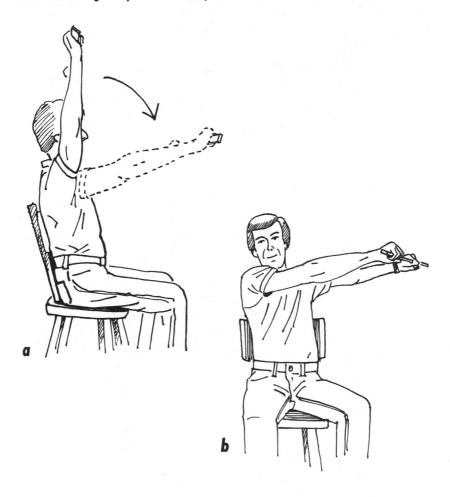

STRAIGHT EDGE, continued

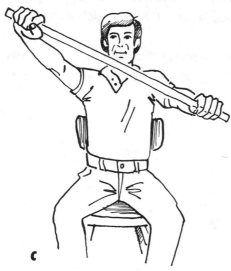

c

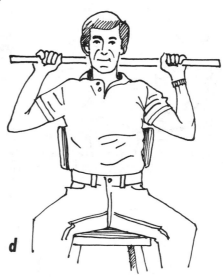

d

WALLFLOWER

Type: Strengthening

Starting position: Stand next to a wall, with the left side of your body about six inches from the wall.

Steps:

1. Lift your right arm out to the side until your forearm is pressing against the wall.
2. Continue to exert pressure for a few seconds at a time.
3. Relax your arm.
4. Turn and repeat the exercise with your left arm.

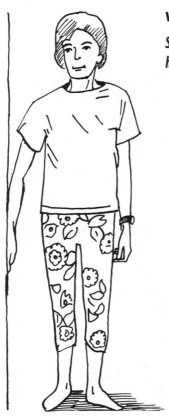

WALLFLOWER

Strengthen your arms, one at a time, by pushing hard against a wall in this isometric exercise.

WEIGHTLIFTER

Type: Strengthening

Starting position: Sit in a straight-back chair or stand at ease, holding one-pound weights.

Steps:
1. Lift the weights straight out in front of you.
2. Lower the weights, then lift them straight out to the sides, to shoulder height if possible.
3. Lower the weights, then try to lift them in back, to a height of about one foot.

PULLEY PULLS

Type: Stretching and strengthening

Starting position: Sit or stand under your pulley rig, with one end of the rope in each hand, arms straight. You can use a real clothesline pulley, hung up for this purpose, or make do with a length of clothesline hung over an open door or on a plastic hook. (Special shoulder exercise pulley rigs that fit standard doors are available by mail order for approximately twenty dollars, see page 50.)

Steps:
1. Pull down with your right hand, letting the motion carry your left hand up as high as possible.
2. Pull down with your left hand, so that your right hand rises on the rope. Experiment with rope length and your grip position to get maximum stretch.
3. Repeat, and return to starting position.

Note: If it's hard for you to hold the rope, make loops of the ends and slip them over your hands. Then you can pull with your forearms.

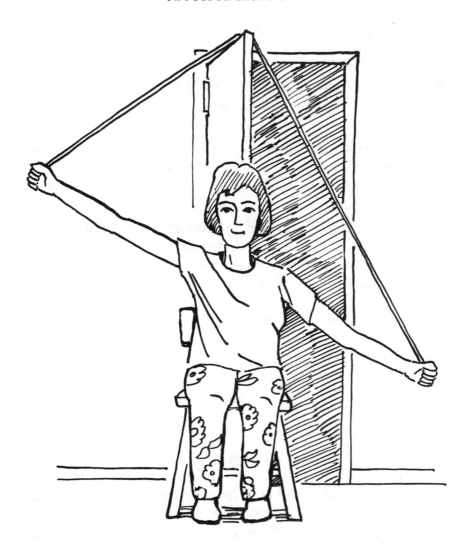

PULLEY PULLS

Work your arms alternately with this simple machine rig, so that each arm allows itself to be raised by the other. This is a shoulder exercise, not a hand exercise, so if you have pain in your hands, feel free to make loops at the ends of your rope and exert the pull force with your forearms.

ROWBOAT

Type: Strengthening

Starting position: Sit in a large rubber tube, with your legs dangling over the rim. Your arms should be free to paddle.

Steps:
1. Using your arms and hands as oars, extend your arms behind you for each stroke and propel yourself across the pool. (Your hands will push the water and send you sailing backward.)
2. Now stroke in the opposite direction, extending your arms ahead of you to begin each stroke. (This time, your hands will pull the water, and you will travel in the direction you are facing.)

If you have access to a swimming pool, try this shoulder-strengthening water exercise. (You need not be a swimmer to attempt it, since it can be done in shallow water.)

PUSH-OFFS

Type: Strengthening

Starting position: Stand facing a wall, with your feet apart and about twelve inches away from the wall. (After you try this exercise, you may find you're more comfortable standing a little closer or a little farther away.) Rest your palms on the wall at about shoulder height. This exercise is a standing push-up.

Steps:
1. Lean in toward the wall as far as possible without touching your forearms to the wall. Keep your legs and back straight. *a*
2. Push yourself back to the starting position. *b*

Note: The farther from the wall you stand, the greater the shoulder effort needed to accomplish the Push-off. As you advance, increase your distance, but don't exceed two feet.

PUSH-OFFS

These stand-up push-ups are easier than the military kind. Nevertheless, they build up strength in the arms and shoulders.

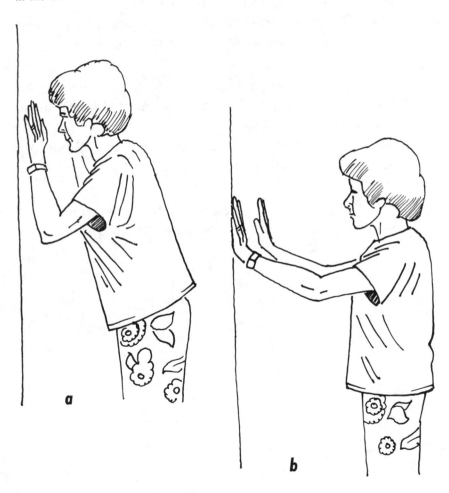

a

b

FAN BELT

Type: Strengthening

Starting position: You may sit or stand in a comfortable position. You will need a rubber exercise belt, or a homemade substitute made from an elasticized belt or bungie cord.

Steps:
1. Slip the belt over your forearms.
2. Spread your forearms as far apart as possible, pushing against the resistance of the exercise belt. **a**
3. Relax.
4. Keeping your arms straight, move the left one up and the right down, again pushing against the resistance of the exercise belt. **b**
5. Move your right arm up and the left down, still pushing against the resistance of the exercise belt.
6. Relax.
7. Take the belt in your hands and pull on it as though you were shooting an arrow, first with your left hand, then your right. **c**

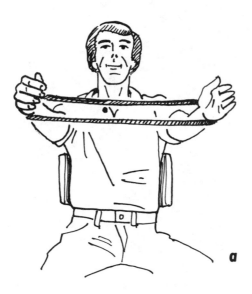

a

FAN BELT

Working your arms against the resistance of an exercise belt or bungie cord can help build shoulder strength.

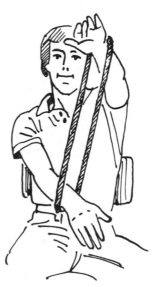

b

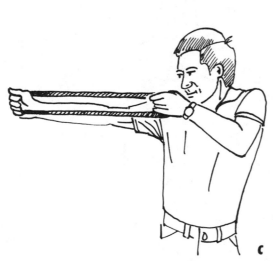

c

CHAPTER 13

Elbow Exercises

How to elbow your way into greater arm strength and range of motion

Many of the exercises recommended for shoulder stretching and strengthening also benefit the elbows, and vice versa. Although the exercises presented in this chapter differ from the shoulder movements in the previous chapter, both sets of exercises tend to benefit both sets of arm joints.

These descriptions call for exercising both elbows together, but of course you may work one elbow at a time if that's easier for you. Ordinary kitchen or living room furniture make ideal gym equipment for these exercises.

ELBOW MACARONI

Type: Stretching

Starting position: You may sit in a straight-back chair or stand at ease, with your arms at your sides.

Steps:
1. Bend your elbow to bring your hand near your shoulder.
2. Move your hand away from your body, down and around to make a circle. Try to keep your upper arm and shoulder still. Return to starting position.
3. Bend your elbow again and circle your hand in the opposite direction, moving it toward your body and around.

WING TUCK

Type: Stretching

Starting position: You may lie on your back, sit in a straight-back chair, or stand at ease, with your arms at your sides, palms facing in.

Steps:
1. Bend and raise your elbows until you can tuck your hands into your armpits. *a*
2. Flap your "wings" down, catching your hands or thumbs under your arms. *b*
3. Raise your elbows again, then return to the starting position.

WING TUCK

Experiment to find the most comfortable way to tuck your hands under your arms—thumbs in or thumbs up. You can achieve the proper stretch either way.

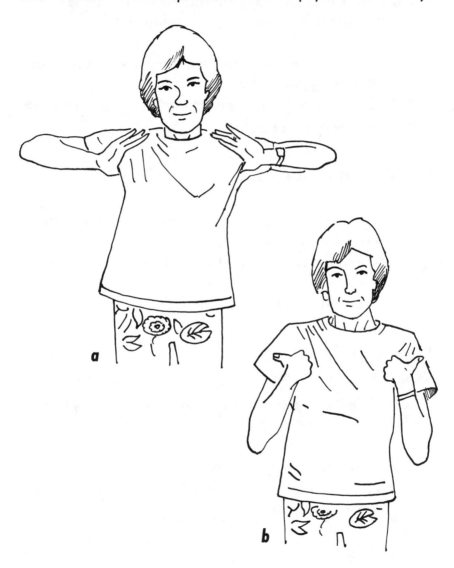

a

b

ELBOW LIMBER-UP #1

Type: Very gentle stretching

Starting position: You may perform this exercise lying in bed, sitting in a straight-back chair, or standing at ease.

Steps:
1. Extend your arms straight out in front at shoulder height, palms facing each other.
2. Bend your elbows and touch your hands to your chest.
3. Reach straight out again.

ELBOW LIMBER-UP #2

Steps:
1. Put your hands on your shoulders so that your elbows point out to the sides.
2. Open your arms, elbows straight, hands extended out as far as you can reach.
3. Return your hands to your shoulders.

ELBOW TWIST

Type: Stretching

Starting position: You may lie in bed, sit in a straight-back chair, or stand at ease.

Steps:
1. Extend your arms out to the sides, palms facing up.
2. Keeping your arms straight, twist your elbows so that your palms face down.

CHOP WOOD

Type: Stretching

Starting position: You may lie on your back or stand at ease.

Steps:

1. Clasp your hands and hold them close to your left shoulder, as though resting an ax there. *a*

2. Gently swing the ax by straightening your elbows and moving your hands toward your right thigh. *b*

3. Raise your clasped hands to your right shoulder, and swing the ax toward your left thigh.

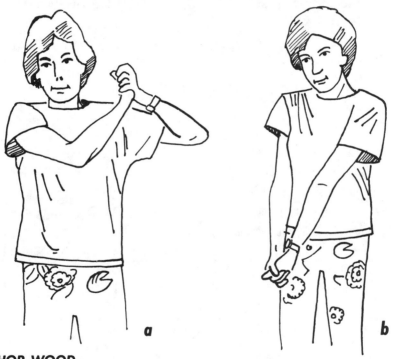

a   *b*

CHOP WOOD

Since you're not really wielding an ax as you swing from shoulder to thigh, you needn't make these movements choppy or jerky. Just aim for maximum stretch.

101

FREE HAND

Type: Stretching

Starting position: You may sit in a straight-back chair or stand at ease, arms at your sides.

Steps:

1. Bend and lift one elbow to shoulder height, leaving your hand dangling free, as though your elbow had been pulled up by a puppet string. (Remember to raise your *elbow*, not your shoulder.)

2. Make circles with your hand, moving your arm below the elbow, first toward the body, then away from the body.

3. Slowly straighten your elbow to return your hand to your side.

4. Repeat with your other elbow.

FREE HAND

Imagine you are a marionette and that the puppeteer has pulled up the string connected to your elbow. This leaves your hand dangling free and swinging in circles.

ELBOW BUILDER

Type: Strengthening

Starting position: Sit in a straight-back chair at a heavy table or desk.

Steps:
1. Put your forearms under the table, with your elbows bent and palms up.
2. Push your forearms up as though trying to lift the table.
3. Hold for a moment, feeling the resistance, then relax.

ALTERNATE ELBOW BUILDER

Type: Strengthening

Starting position: You may sit or stand, with your arms at your sides.

Steps:
1. Cross your right forearm over your left, both palms facing up.
2. Press down with your right forearm and up with your left, without moving your arms in either direction.
3. Hold for a moment, feeling the resistance of one arm against the other.
4. Repeat with your left forearm over your right.

CHAPTER 14

Wrist Exercises

*How to gain strength and flexibility from a twist of
the wrist*

Since most wrist exercises can be done from virtually any
starting position—lying in bed, sitting in a chair, or standing
at ease—we won't specify a position unless we have to. The
only essential requirement is that you allow your wrists
enough room to move.

In most cases, the choice is yours whether you wish to
exercise both wrists together or work one at a time.

If you have severely affected wrists that have been set at a
new angle by arthritis, please be careful to exercise *against* the
drift only. Your goal is to regain lost ground.

WRIST ASSIST

Type: Very gentle stretching

Steps:

1. Using your left hand to help the right, gently bend your right wrist so that your right hand drops forward. **a**

2. Bend your right wrist the opposite way, so that your left hand is raised. **b**

3. Repeat the movements to exercise the left wrist.

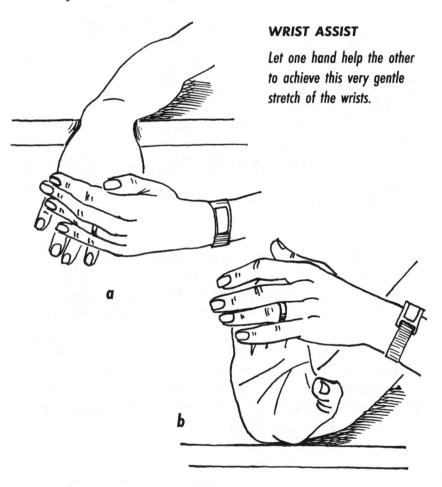

WRIST ASSIST

Let one hand help the other to achieve this very gentle stretch of the wrists.

WRIST ROTATOR

Type: Stretching

Steps:

1. Rest your forearm and hand on a flat surface. Rotate your wrist so that your hand slides in a clockwise direction as far as it can go. Try not to lift your fingers, or move your elbow, but just work your wrist. *a*

2. Hold for a moment, feeling the stretch, then rotate your wrist to make your hand slide counterclockwise. *b*

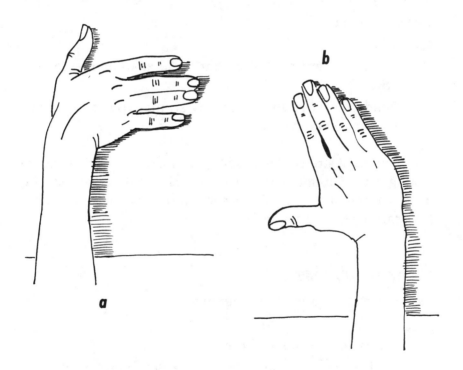

WRIST ROTATOR

Slowly swivel each hand from side to side, swiveling your wrist. Your hand should move like a windshield wiper on slow speed.

TWIST

Type: Gentle stretching

Steps:
1. Rest your forearm and hand with your palm down on a flat surface. Twist your wrist so that your palm is turned toward the ceiling.
2. Twist back so that your palm rests on the flat surface.

STOP AND GO

Type: Stretching

Steps:
1. Bend your wrist to raise your hand as though signaling "Stop."
2. Bend your wrist the other way so that your hand drops forward as far as it can go.

Note: For extra stretch, try the Stop and Go with your forearm resting on a flat surface, and your wrist at its edge. As you make each motion, use the other hand to push your wrist a little farther than it wants to go.

SWAYING PALMS

Type: Stretching and strengthening

Steps:
1. Clasp your hands in front.
2. Push your right palm against the left, bending the left wrist back.
3. Push your left palm against the right, bending the right wrist back.

FIGURE EIGHTS

Type: Stretching

Starting position: You may rest your forearm on a flat surface, with your wrist extending free over the edge. Another way is to extend your arms, and pretend you are conducting an orchestra. You can also let your arms hang at your sides, or bend them at the elbows.

Steps:
1. Trace a figure-eight pattern in the air with your hand, so that your wrist executes twists and turns through its full range of motion. Your fingers may assume any relaxed position you like.
2. As you become comfortable with this exercise, exaggerate the motion by bending your wrist more sharply through these twists and turns.

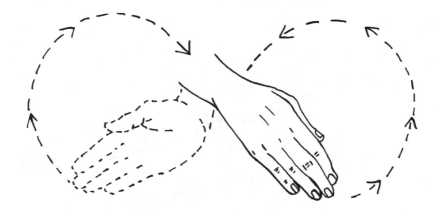

FIGURE EIGHTS

Trace the pattern of a figure eight in the air. The many twists and turns will put your wrists through their full range of motion.

WRIST BUILDER

Type: Stretching and strengthening

Steps:

1. Hold a light saucepan out as though trying to catch drips from a leak.

2. Using your wrist to make the motion, twist the saucepan over as though dumping it out.

WRIST RISE

Type: Strengthening

Steps:

1. Sitting at a table, reach your hand under it, with your palm facing the floor.

2. Press the back of your hand against the table, feeling the pressure in your wrist. *a*

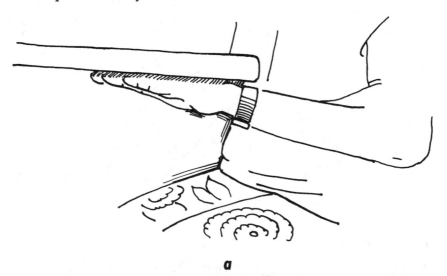

a

Variation:

1. Put your left hand on the surface of the table, palm down.

2. With the heel of your right hand, push down on your left hand while simultaneously trying to raise the left hand against the pressure. **b** Here again, motion is not the goal; developing strength through isometric exercise is.

3. Repeat with the left hand over the right.

WRIST RISE

Here's another way to strengthen your wrists by trying to lift each one against the opposing pressure of a table, or your other hand.

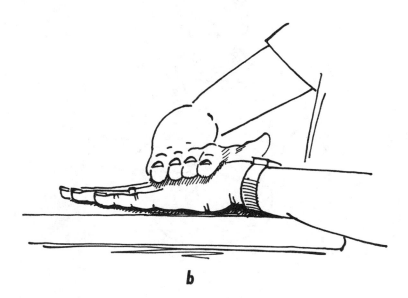

b

PRAYING HANDS

Type: Strengthening

Steps:

1. Put the palms of your hands together as though in prayer, with your elbows out and wrists bent at right angles.
2. Press your palms together, allowing no movement in either direction.
3. Hold, feeling the push in your wrists.

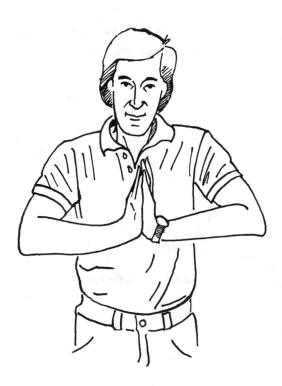

PRAYING HANDS

Although no movement is visible in this isometric exercise, the pressure of one hand against the other safely strengthens the wrists.

CHAPTER 15

Hand and Finger Exercises

How to help prevent hand and finger deformities with exercises that preserve your manual dexterity

Hand and finger exercises can fit into the busiest schedule, virtually anywhere. Since they often involve fine movements that require effort and concentration, you may find that you prefer to exercise one hand at a time. Your hands are well worth the individual attention, as each one contains fifteen joints—not counting the wrist!

If you have rheumatoid arthritis, you may have one or another of the hand and finger deformities that frequently accompany this disease. The deformities may result from weakness in the muscles and ligaments that allow the joints to bend at odd angles. In ulnar deviation, for example, the fingers appear tilted sideways at the knuckles, and thus seem

113

to slant away from the thumbs. If you have this condition, avoid any exercises that might aggravate the drift. Try to exercise in the opposite direction only, in an effort to correct the deformity.

The swan's neck and boutonniere deformities involve the joints closest to the fingertips and the middle joints of the fingers, freezing them in characteristic positions. In swan's neck, the fingertip bends down, following the normal direction of motion, but the middle joint bends up, as though broken. This gives the finger the appearance of a swan's arched neck. The boutonniere deformity is just the opposite: the fingertip bends up, while the middle joint bends down. Exercise can help prevent and sometimes even correct these deformities. For example, the Okay All Around and Typist's Warm-up exercises support normal motions of the fingers, and the Squeeze Play exercise strengthens the muscles, ligaments, and tendons of the hands.

People with osteoarthritis may develop excess bony growths in their finger joints. These are called Heberden's nodes when they occur at the joints nearest the fingertips, and Bouchard's nodes when they occur at the middle joints. The nodes may cause pain, swelling, or redness as they develop, but most discomfort soon subsides. In any case, the nodes need not limit hand function to any great extent. Regular exercise will make sure of that!

Many people find that exercise goes more swimmingly in water. All of the following movements can be done in a sink or basin of warm water. (You'll need to modify the Wall Walker a bit, by walking up the sides of the basin, and do the Finger Curls without raising your hand in greeting.) If you decide to immerse your hands, then arrange your exercise space so that you can keep the rest of your body comfortable while you give your hands a workout.

FINGER SPREAD

Type: Gentle stretching

Steps:
1. With your palm resting on a flat surface, spread your fingers as widely apart as possible.
2. Slowly draw your fingers together again, still keeping your palm flat.

TYPIST'S WARM-UP

Type: Full stretching

Steps:
1. Make fists of both hands.
2. Relax your hands.
3. Wiggle your fingers up and down.
4. Circle your wrists.
5. Rub your hands together, as though you were rubbing lotion on them.

FINGER LIFTS

Type: Stretching

Steps:
1. With your hand resting on a flat surface, lift your thumb as high as you can and then rest it.
2. Lift your index finger as high as you can, without raising any of the other fingers, and then rest it.
3. Lift your middle finger in turn, then rest it.
4. This is the hardest part for most people: lift your ring finger as high as you can, and then rest it.
5. Lift your little finger, then rest it.

OKAY ALL AROUND

Type: Gentle stretching

Steps:

1. Make the "okay" sign by joining the tips of your index finger and thumb. Hold for a few seconds, keeping your other fingers as straight as you comfortably can. *a*

2. Straighten your index finger and join the tip of your middle finger to your thumb. *b*

3. After straightening your middle finger, join your ring finger and thumb. *c*

4. In the same fashion, touch the tip of your little finger to your thumb. *d*

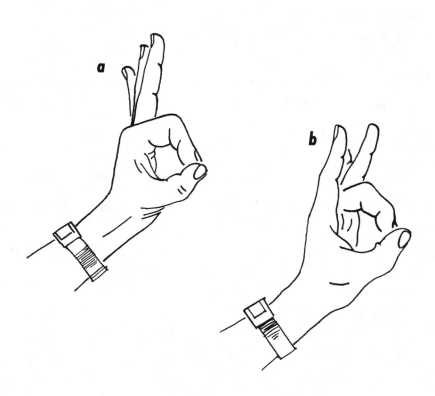

Note: You can add strengthening to the stretch of this exercise by pressing your fingertips lightly together for a few seconds each time you join your thumb to another finger. Since the joints don't move with the pressure, this is an isometric exercise.

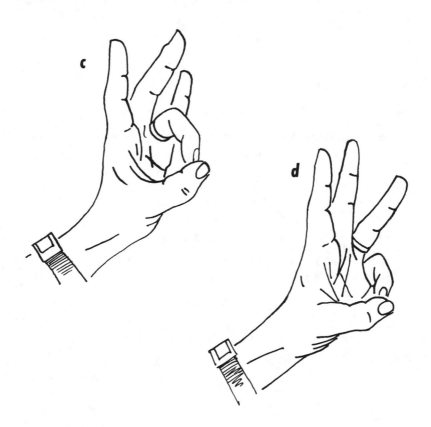

OKAY ALL AROUND

Stretch all your fingers with these variations on the "okay" theme. Make the "okay" sign with each one in turn.

Strengthen your fingers, too, by pressing the thumb and each finger together with a little extra pressure.

FINGER PUSH-UPS

Type: Strengthening

Steps: Follow the same steps as for Finger Lifts above, but move each finger against pressure. You can do this by sliding your hand under your buttocks in bed, by pushing against the underside of a desk or table, or by exerting counterpressure with your other hand.

WALL WALKER

Type: Stretching

Starting position: You may stand or sit about two feet away from a wall, with your left side to the wall, arms at your sides.

Steps:
1. Let your left hand slowly "walk" up the wall, as though your fingers were the legs of an insect. *a*
2. "Walk" above shoulder level if you can, but try not to raise your shoulder or lean away from the wall. "Let your fingers do the walking." *b*
3. Turn and "walk" your right hand.

Note: This exercise is also included in the Shoulder section, as it benefits those joints as well.

WALL WALKER

Walk your fingers up a wall, letting them do all the work. Think of them as a five-legged insect that found its way into your house.

Send your fingers up as high as they can go, without raising your shoulder to help them and without leaning away from the wall.

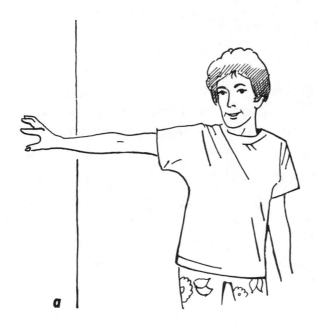

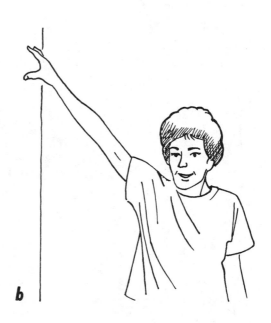

FINGER SLIDES

Type: Stretching

Steps:

1. With your hand resting on a flat surface, slide your index finger as far as it will go toward your thumb.
2. Still keeping your hand flat, move the middle finger to meet your index finger. *a*
3. Slide the ring finger over, too. *b*

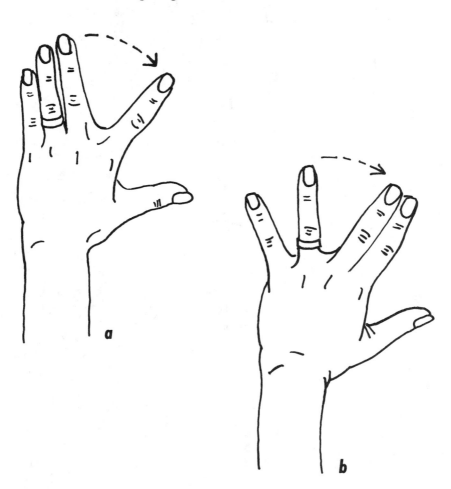

4. Your little finger has no doubt followed the movement of your other fingers. Let it go the rest of the way now. **c**

5. Beginning with the little finger, slide your fingers one by one away from your thumb. **d**

FINGER SLIDES

It takes control and concentration to stretch your fingers by moving each one individually in this fashion. The real challenge comes in holding the rest still while one moves.

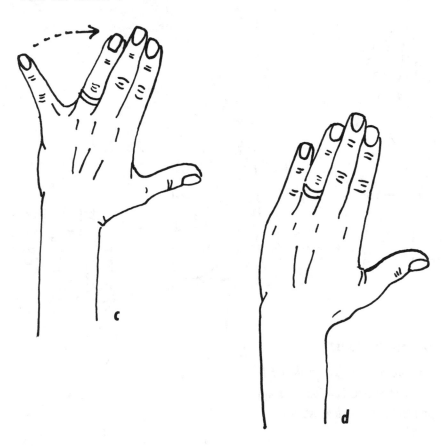

THUMB WRESTLE

Type: Stretching

Steps:

1. With your hand open and fingers straight, extend your thumb away from your other fingers as far as you can. **a**

2. Move your thumb forward so it is perpendicular to your palm. **b**

3. Reach your thumb across your palm and try to touch your little finger. **c**

4. Circle your thumb in the opposite direction.

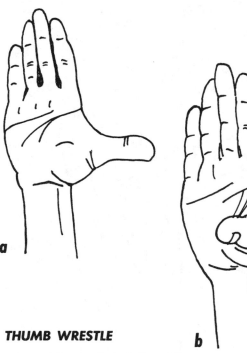

a

THUMB WRESTLE

Put your thumbs through their full range of motion by acting out this prelude to a thumb-wrestling match.

b

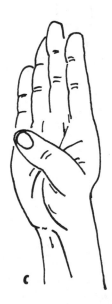

c

FINGER CURLS

Type: Difficult stretching

Steps:

1. Hold your hand up, as though greeting someone, with your fingers as straight as possible.
2. Slowly curl the index finger by bending the joint nearest the fingertip *a*, then the middle joint *b*, until the tip of your index finger touches the uppermost part of your palm. You may move the finger with your other hand, if need be.
3. Uncurl your index finger.
4. Attempt the same maneuvers with the middle finger.
5. Curl and uncurl the ring finger the same way.
6. Curl and uncurl the little finger.
7. Moving all four fingers simultaneously, curl and uncurl them.

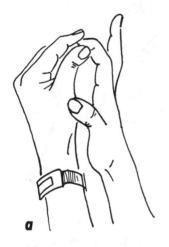 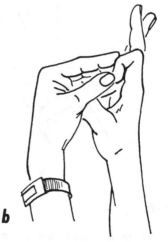

a   b

FINGER CURLS

One joint at a time, bend and then straighten each finger. You'll definitely need the help of the opposite hand to accomplish this unusual movement.

FINGER SKIDS

Type: Strengthening

Steps:

Follow the same steps you did for Finger Slides, but use the tip of your index finger to resist, for a few seconds, the movement of each finger.

Note: Since the tendency in rheumatoid arthritis is for the fingers to slant away from the thumb, it's best to perform this strengthening exercise *toward* the thumb.

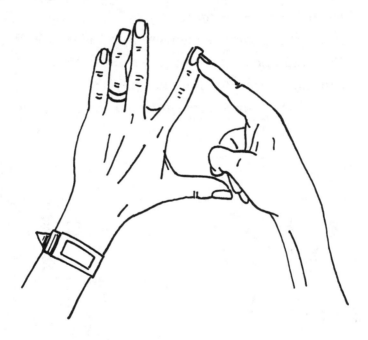

FINGER SKIDS

By adding resistance from the opposite hand, the Finger Slide stretch changes into the Finger Skid strengthener.

If your hands are turned outward, as is often the case in rheumatoid arthritis, exercise in only one direction—against the drift of the deformity.

SQUEEZE PLAY

Type: Strengthening

Steps:

1. Squeeze and work a small rubber ball or therapeutic putty in each hand.

FINGER STRAIGHTENERS

Type: Corrective (The goal of this exercise is to help straighten fingers affected by swan's neck and boutonniere deformities.)

Steps:

1. Rest your left hand, palm down, on a table top.
2. Flatten your hand and fingers as much as you can.
3. Using the heel of your right hand to exert pressure, gently push the left finger joints flat.
4. Repeat the steps for flattening with your right hand.

CHAPTER 16

Back Exercises

How to exercise away back pain by stretching and strengthening your abdominal muscles

The exercises in this section are called back exercises, but as you'll see, the place you really feel them is in your gut. Performing them faithfully will stretch and strengthen the abdominal muscles you need to maintain good posture and a normal level of activity. As a bonus, you'll probably wind up with a flatter tummy.

We recommend the starred exercises as an essential part of every exercise regimen. Even if you feel no pain or stiffness in your back, you will no doubt find that these maneuvers increase your general muscle tone and flexibility. They will also help keep back pain at bay.

Probably the most common, serious mistake people make with regard to back exercise is attempting sit-ups with the legs straight. This position is risky for the back. You can achieve the same good effects—better effects, in fact, because you won't be using your hip muscles as much—by keeping your knees bent as you sit up and lie back down. Another approach, as you'll see, is to reverse the usual order by performing Sit-downs instead of Sit-ups.

Anyone can have back pain, with or without arthritis. Even people who know they have arthritis may suffer back pain from other causes. Given this possibility, get prompt treatment for any back pain that comes on suddenly and sharply. This is likely the result of a muscle strain, and may require a couple of days' rest to clear up. If the pain in your back travels down your legs, it may be due to a problem with one of your discs—the cushioning tissue between the verte-brae of the spine. Bulging discs can press against spinal nerves, often bringing on a tingling or burning sensation or extreme weakness in the legs. The same symptoms can result from the normal flattening of the discs that comes with age, or from the bone spurs that sprout on the vertebrae as a result of osteoarthritis. Check with your doctor. Whatever the cause of the discomfort, exercise—especially gentle stretching and strengthening—invariably plays a role in any back-pain treat-ment plan.

KNEE TO CHEST (*)

Type: Stretching

Starting position: Lie on your back, knees bent and feet flat, arms relaxed at your sides.

Steps:
1. Lift your right knee toward your chest as far as you can. *a*
2. Lower knee to and through starting position, so your right leg is extended straight on the bed (or floor). *b*

3. Wobble your leg to relax the muscles.
4. Return to starting position.
5. Repeat for your left leg.

Advanced addition: If you can move your knee easily toward your chest, try pulling it with your hands to bring it still closer.

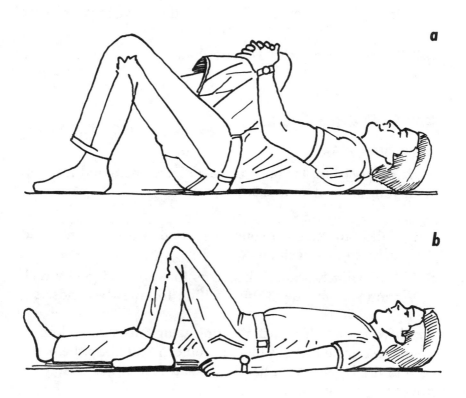

KNEE TO CHEST

Pulling the knee to the chest gives the lower back a gentle stretch. You'll feel the curve in your lower back straighten out as you do this.

129

⌐ TILT (*)

Type: Stretching and strengthening

Starting position: Lie on your back with your knees bent so you can keep your feet flat. Leave your arms relaxed at your sides.

Steps:
1. Tighten your buttocks and pull in your abdominal muscles. Exhale as you do this. The movement will cave in your abdomen and flatten out the curve in your lower back.

2. Relax your muscles as you inhale.

KNEE TO CHEST ROCK

Type: Stretching

Starting position: Lie on your back, knees bent and feet flat, with your arms at your sides.

Steps:
1. Pull both knees to your chest, one at a time, and hold them in this position. *a*

2. Curl your head and shoulders forward and gently rock from side to side in this position for a few seconds. *b*

Simplified version: If you can't bring your knees very close to your chest, raise them as high as you can and grasp the backs of your thighs with your hands, instead of trying to clasp your knees in your arms. *a*

Advanced addition: Bring both knees up together and clasp your arms around them. *b*

KNEE TO CHEST ROCK

Depending on your degree of flexibility, you can achieve this rocking motion by grasping your legs at different places.

If you are new to exercise, make this easy on yourself by grasping the backs of your thighs; that's the easiest way. Holding your knees is the intermediate position, while clasping your arms around both knees gives the greatest stretch and is the most difficult way to approach this exercise.

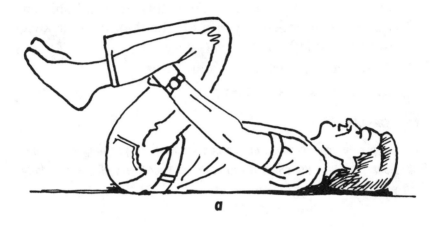

a

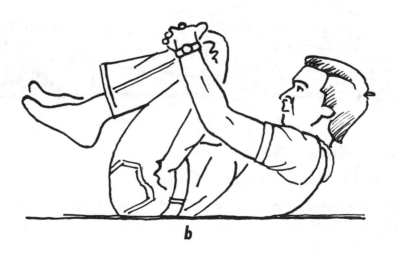

b

KNEE DROPS

Type: Stretching

Starting position: Lie on your back with your knees bent and feet flat.

Steps:
1. Keeping your knees together, drop both of them to the left as far as you can. Try to keep both shoulders touching the bed (floor) as you do this. Your right hip and buttock will necessarily rise off the floor as your knees drop to the left.
2. Return to the starting position.
3. Drop both knees to the right.

KNEE DROPS

Try to keep both your shoulders on the bed (or floor) as you drop your knees first to one side, then the other. If you can't get your knees all the way down, don't worry. You'll build up to that in time.

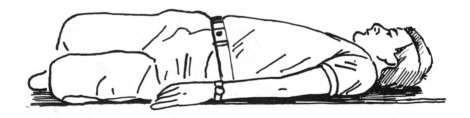

BENT-KNEE SIT-UPS

Type: Stretching and strengthening

Starting position: Lie on your back, knees bent and feet flat, arms relaxed at your sides.

Steps:

1. Exhaling, pull in your abdominals and raise the upper part of your body toward your knees. You need not come very far up (just far enough to see your navel), and you may lead with your outstretched arms.

2. Hold the position, but don't hold your breath, for a few seconds. Be conscious of breathing in and out.

3. Inhaling, relax your muscles slowly as you lower your head and shoulders.

Advanced addition: Instead of leading with your arms, try doing this exercise with your arms folded across your chest.

BENT-KNEE SIT-UPS

Sit-ups from a bent-knee position give just as good a workout to the abdominal muscles as the old straight-knee sit-ups you learned in school. More important, they are much safer for the back. While steady breathing is important during any exercise, you'll get a real boost here if you exhale as you sit up, then inhale as you lie back down.

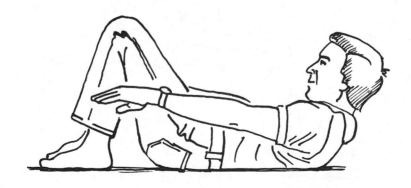

133

SIT-DOWNS

Type: Stretching and strengthening

Starting position: You may sit on an exercise bench or the edge of your bed. Fold your arms across your chest, or extend them out in front of you.

Steps:

1. Exhaling, use your abdominal muscles to lean your body backward several inches—about as far as you lift up for a sit-up. (As you advance, you may be able to lean farther back.)

2. Hold the position, but don't hold your breath, for a count of three. Be conscious of breathing in and out.

3. Inhaling, return to a straight sitting posture and relax your muscles.

SIT-DOWNS

These reverse sit-ups provide yet another way to stretch and strengthen the abdominals.

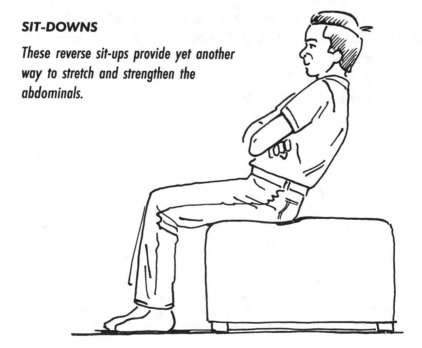

CAT STRETCH

Type: Full stretching

Starting position: Get down on the floor on all fours with your back flat and your weight evenly distributed. **a**

Steps:

1. Slide your hands forward, letting your elbows bend and touch the floor. **b**
2. Lower your head and raise your rear end.
3. Smoothly sink back on your haunches, so that you are almost sitting on your ankles. (Your elbows will straighten out as you do this step.) **c**
4. Return to the starting position. **d**
5. Drop your head and pull in your abdominals to curve your back like a Halloween cat. **e**
6. Relax your muscles and roll your head back. **f**

a

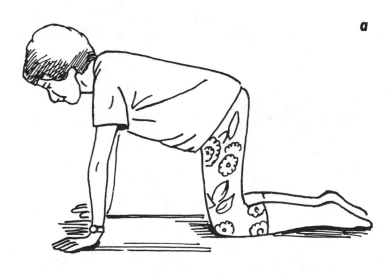

135

CAT STRETCH, continued

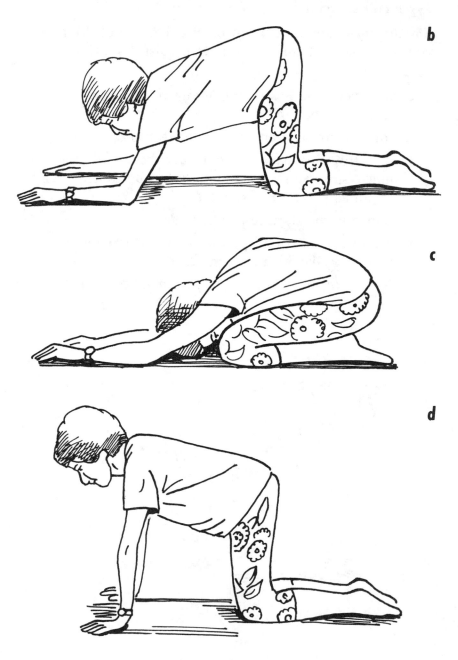

b

c

d

CAT STRETCH

The several steps of this exercise mimic the motions cats make with their supple spines as they awaken from one of their famed catnaps.

The completed series gives you a full yet gentle stretch in all directions.

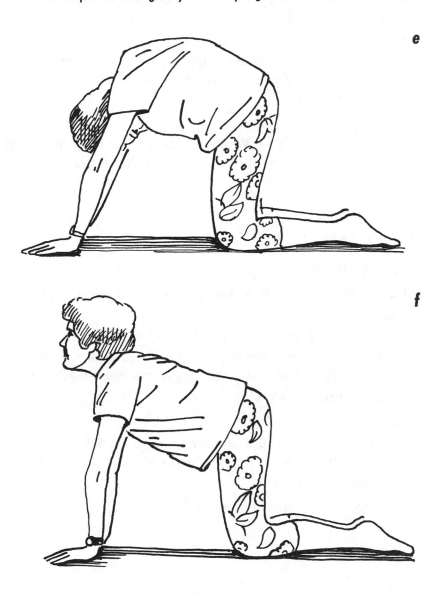

e

f

ROLLER BLADES

Type: Stretching

Starting position: You may stand in a comfortable position or sit on the edge of a chair. (Steps 1 and 2 may also be done while lying down.)

Steps:
1. Squeeze your shoulders together for a few seconds in an effort to make your shoulder blades meet in the middle of your back.
2. Relax.
3. Again, try to make your shoulder blades meet, this time by pushing your elbows together behind you.

TWISTS AND TURNS

Type: Stretching

Starting position: Sit in a straight-back chair or stand at ease.

Steps:
1. Rest your hands on your hips and lean the top of your body to the left. Try not to bend forward as you do this. Also, try to keep your feet, legs, and hips steady. *a*
2. Straighten up slowly.
3. Repeat these motions to the right.
4. Twist the upper half of your body to the left, as though trying to see behind you. Keep your lower body still. *b*
5. Return to face front.
6. Repeat these motions to the right.

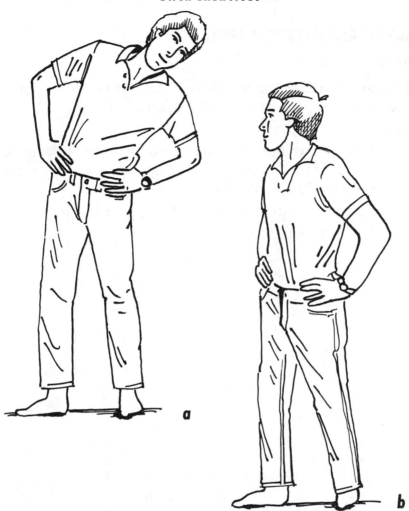

TWISTS AND TURNS

Give yourself a maximum sideways stretch with these maneuvers. Try very hard not to bend forward as you lean to the right or left.

For the second part of this stretch, twist your body to the side to find out what's going on behind you.

BACK AGAINST THE WALL

Type: Strengthening

Starting position: You may sit in a straight-back chair, or on the floor with your back literally against the wall.

Steps:

1. Exhale as you press the upper part of your back against the chair back or wall—as though you could push your shoulder blades through it.

2. Hold the position without holding your breath.

3. Inhale as you relax.

CHAPTER 17

Hip
Exercises

How to perform effective hip exercises standing,
sitting, or lying down—even in the pool

The hips boast a wide range of normal motion that enables us to do everything from walk forward to slide sideways on a bench—not to mention pedal backwards on a bicycle and bend down to tie a shoelace. Individual exercises stretch and strengthen different muscles that control the hips. In your exercise program, you will want to incorporate at least one exercise for each type and direction of hip motion. For example, a beginner's program might include the Leg Spread, the Straight Leg-ups, the Simple Knee Cross, and the Liftback. Each one emphasizes a different movement.

Many exercises for the back also benefit the hips, such as the Knee to Chest. Sometimes, people with low back pain

ve trouble attempting certain hip exercises, and need anoth-
r way to accomplish the same stretch. For example, the
Simple Knee Cross is a variation of the Knee Cross intended
specifically for people suffering from back pain.

LEG SPREAD

Type: Stretching

Starting position: Lie on your back with your legs out
straight.

Steps:
1. Spread your legs as far apart as you can to give your hips
   a sideways stretch.
2. Bring your legs back together.

Caution: If you have back pain, move one leg at a time, keeping
the inactive leg bent at the knee.

Advanced addition: Lift your legs slightly before spreading
them, so they glide through the air instead of sliding on the
bed (or floor).

Note: You can turn this stretch into a strengthening exercise by
looping an exercise belt over your ankles, calves, or thighs and
then spreading your legs against the resistance of the belt.

LEG ROLL

Type: Stretching

Starting position: Lie on your back, with your right knee bent
and your left leg straight.

Steps:
1. Flex your left foot so that your toes point to the ceiling.

2. Rotate your left leg counterclockwise so that your toes point to the side, away from your body. (Feel the twist in your hip.) *a*

3. Rotate your left leg in the opposite direction, pointing your toes toward the ceiling again, and then toward your right side. *b*

4. Relax your left foot.

5. Switch position so your right leg is extended and your left leg is bent at the knee.

6. Repeat the rotation movements with your right leg.

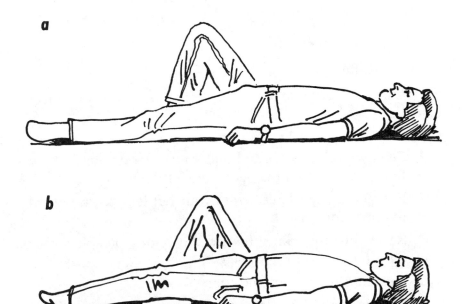

a

b

LEG ROLL

Make your hip do the work of rotating your leg first out, then in. Think of it as a log roll!

143

₹AIGHT LEG-UPS

Type: Stretching and strengthening

Starting position: Lie on your back, with your knees bent and feet flat, arms relaxed at your sides.

Steps:
1. Straighten your right leg so it lies flat.
2. Lift your right leg, keeping your knee straight, as high as you can.
3. Lower your leg slowly.
4. Bend your knee to return to the starting position.
5. Repeat the movements with your left leg.

SIMPLE KNEE CROSS

Type: Stretching

Starting position: Lie on your left side, with your legs extended.

Steps:
1. Bend your right knee and pull it up toward your body so that your right foot is near your left knee. *a*
2. Press your right knee across your left leg, down toward the floor (or bed). *b*
3. Raise your right knee toward the ceiling, keeping your right foot on your left knee. *c*
4. Return to the starting position.
5. Turn to your right side and repeat the movement with your left leg.

SIMPLE KNEE CROSS

One knee crosses the other in this maneuver, but the hips do most of the work and get most of the stretch.

As you raise and lower your knee, picture the gentle motion of a butterfly's wing.

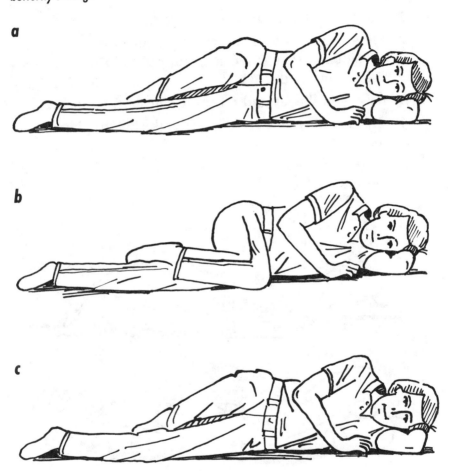

145

KNEE CROSS

Type: Stretching

Starting position: Lie on your back, with your knees bent and feet flat, arms relaxed at your sides.

Steps:

1. Cross your left thigh over the right. *a*
2. Press your legs together and tip your knees toward the left side as far as you can. (Your right hip will naturally rise as you do this.) *b*
3. Raise your knees and return to the starting position.
4. Repeat with your right thigh over the left, tipping toward the right.

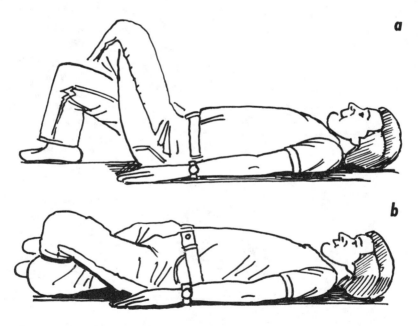

a

b

KNEE CROSS

This is a more difficult way to cross the knees—and stretch the hips. Remember, you can't be expected to make a touch-down the first time you try this.

LATERAL LEG-UPS

Type: Strengthening

Starting position: Lie on your right side, with your legs straight. Prop your left hand in front of your body for support.

Steps:
1. Lift your left leg as high as you can, keeping it straight.
2. Hold it at the height you reached for several seconds.
3. Lower it gently.
4. Repeat.
5. Turn over and repeat the movement with your right leg.

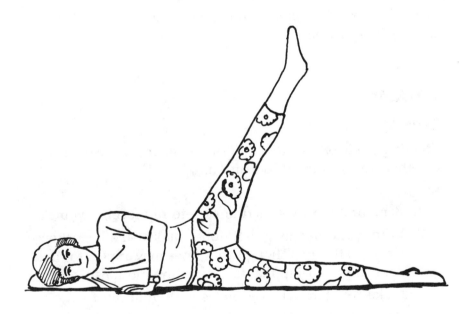

LATERAL LEG-UPS

Raising your legs straight up from the side builds hip strength. Lift each as far as you comfortably can. To keep your balance as you go through this exercise, prop your upper hand in front of you.

FORCED MARCH

Type: Stretching

Starting position: Stand in a comfortable position. You may use the back of a chair to lean on for support if need be.

Steps:
1. Bend and raise your left knee as high as you can, as though you were taking a step in an exaggerated military march.
2. Lower your left knee so your foot is on the floor where it started. (No need to march forward.)
3. Repeat the movement with your right knee.

Note: This exercise appears in the Knee section, as it benefits those joints as well.

CANCAN

Type: Stretching

Starting position: Stand comfortably, giving yourself a chair or other sturdy support to lean on.

Steps:
1. Bend and raise your left knee—to hip level, if you can.
2. With your dangling left foot, make small clockwise circles in the air. (Though your knee may appear to circle, it's really your hip that facilitates the motions.)
3. Make counterclockwise circles with your left foot.
4. Return to the starting position.
5. Repeat the movements with your right knee and foot.

Note: This exercise also appears in the Knee section, as it benefits those joints as well.

CANCAN

Circle your raised foot in clockwise, then counterclockwise circles in the air—as those famed chorus lines of dancers did.

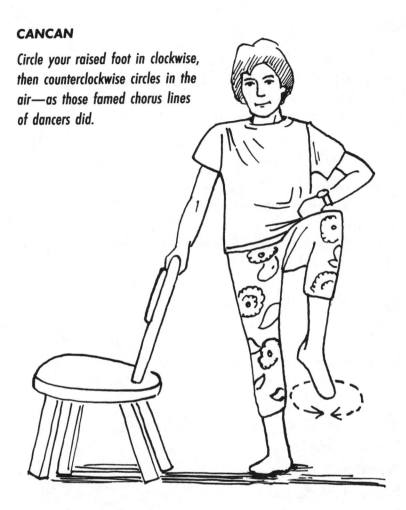

HULA HOOP

Type: Stretching

Starting position: Stand in a comfortable position.

Steps:
1. Slowly and gently, swivel your hips in circles to the left, as though you were trying to twirl a hula hoop.
2. Swivel your hips to the right.

LIFTBACKS

Type: Stretching

Starting position: You may lie face down or stand facing a chair that you can lean on for support. The standing position works better for people with back pain.

Steps:

1. Raise your right leg behind you as far as you can.
2. Lower your right leg.
3. Repeat with the left leg.

Note: If you stand during this exercise, make sure to lean your upper body forward to avoid arching your back.

LEG LIFTS

Type: Stretching

Starting position: Stand to the side of a chair that you can lean on for support.

Steps:

1. Raise your left leg straight out in front of you.
2. Lower your left leg.
3. Repeat with the right leg.
4. Turn to face the chair support.
5. Lift your left leg out to the side and then lower it.
6. Lift and then lower your right leg out to the side.

SWORDPLAY

Type: Stretching

Starting position: Stand facing the back of a chair, with both your hands on it for support.

Steps:

1. Move your right foot far to the side and put your weight on it. Bend your right knee as far as you can, keeping your left leg straight.
2. Hold for a few seconds to feel the stretch.
3. Return to the starting position.
4. Make the same sort of fencer's lunge to the left side, keeping your right leg straight.

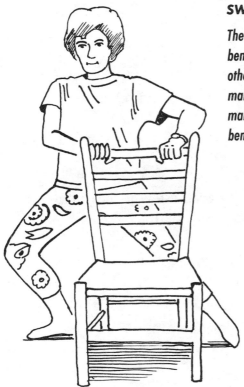

SWORDPLAY

The stretch in this exercise comes from bending one leg and extending the other as though fighting a duel with make-believe swords. You need not make a sudden lunge to reap the benefits.

HIP WALKOUT

Type: Stretching and strengthening

Starting position: Stand where you have room to walk.

Steps:
1. Walk a few steps.
2. Turn out your feet, as Charlie Chaplin used to do, and walk a bit more.
3. Turn your feet towards each other, pigeon-toed, and walk on.

THE SQUEEZE

Type: Strengthening

Starting position: You may do this exercise lying down, sitting, or standing.

Steps:
1. Squeeze your buttocks together as tightly as you can.
2. Hold for a moment, then release, and relax.

HIP STRENGTHENER

Type: Strengthening

Starting position: Stand with a wall a few inches from your left side and a support chair to your right.

Steps:
1. Raise your left leg to the side, so that your leg is fully pressed against the wall.
2. Keep pushing your left leg against the wall's resistance.
3. Relax and return to the starting position.
4. Turn and repeat the motion with your right leg.

If you have access to a warm swimming pool or a large hot tub, you can incorporate the following water exercises into your regimen of hip exercises.

SCISSOR KICK

Type: Stretching

Starting position: Sit on the pool steps or the hot tub bench with both legs extended straight out in front.

Steps:
1. Spread your legs as far apart as you can.
2. Bring your legs together and scissor-cross them left over right.
3. Spread them far apart again.
4. Make a scissor-cross with your right leg over your left.

FLUTTER KICK

Type: Strengthening

Starting position: Face the side of the pool and hold on to it.

Steps:
1. Raise your legs behind you.
2. Slowly kick your legs up and down as though you were swimming.

LEG CIRCLES

Type: Stretching and strengthening

Starting position: Stand in the water, with your left arm out to the side, holding the edge of the pool.

Steps:

1. Raise your right leg, and make a large, slow clockwise circle.

2. Still using your right leg, complete a large, slow, counter-clockwise circle.

3. Turn and repeat the circles with your left leg.

JUMPING JACKS

Type: Strengthening

Starting position: Stand in the water with your hands on your hips.

Steps:

1. Letting the water help buoy you, jump into a legs-apart position.

2. Jump and bring your feet together again.

CHAPTER 18

Knee Exercises

How to bend and straighten the weight-bearing joints of the knees to best advantage

When functioning properly, the knees support us through a remarkable number of daily activities, absorbing the shock of walking and stair-climbing. Unfortunately, the hinge joints of the knees also are common targets for both osteoarthritis and rheumatoid arthritis.

Exercising the muscles that control the knee's opening and closing movements is the best way to maintain function and flexibility. You'll notice that many of the exercises in this section concentrate on perfecting the knee's ability to straighten all the way. It's easy to understand the importance of these maneuvers when you remember that the knee becomes unevenly stressed if it tries to do everything from a half-bent position, and such stress eventually leads to further damage.

Some of the exercises in this section have been borrowed from the chapters on back and hip exercises, but most are specifically designed to straighten, stretch, and strengthen the knees, which you may work singly or together.

KNEE TO CHEST PLUS

Type: Stretching

Starting position: Lie on your back, knees bent and feet flat, arms relaxed at your sides.

Steps:
1. Lift your right knee toward your chest as far as you can. *a*
2. Lower your knee to and through the starting position, so your right leg is extended straight on the bed (or floor). *b*
3. Wobble your leg to relax the muscles.
4. Return to the starting position by bending your knee and sliding your foot back toward your body.
5. Continue sliding your foot back, bringing it as close to your buttocks as you can. (You may pull your foot with your hand.) Hold this position briefly. *c*
6. Return to the starting position.
7. Repeat for your left leg.

Advanced addition: If you can move your knee easily toward your chest, try pulling it with your hands to bring it still closer.

KNEE TO CHEST PLUS

Knee workouts are all about bending and straightening. This extra step in the basic Knee to Chest exercise—bringing the heel right up to the buttock—adds a good knee bend to an otherwise excellent back stretch.

a

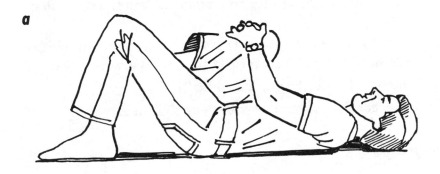

b

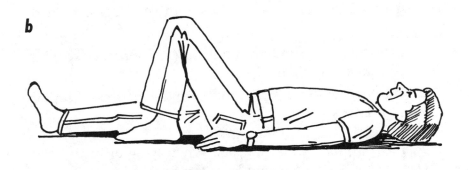

c

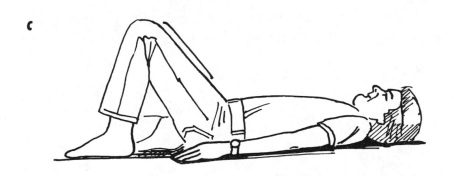

KNEE PUSH

Type: Stretching

Starting position: Lie on your back, with your knees bent.

Steps:

1. Straighten your left leg so it rests full length on the floor (or bed).
2. Try to straighten your left knee even beyond straight— as though you could push it to bend the wrong way.
3. Return to the starting position.
4. Repeat the movement with your right leg.

KNEE PRESS

Type: Stretching and strengthening

Starting position: Lie on your back with your legs extended.

Steps:

1. Press your heels into the mattress (or floor mat), keeping your knees straight.
2. Turn over and press your toes into the mattress, keeping your knees straight.

Precaution for people with back pain: When lying on your back, press one heel at a time, and keep the resting leg bent at the knee.

When lying face down, put a small pillow under your abdomen as a support for your lower back.

KNEE KICKS

Type: Stretching

Starting position: Lie on your back with your knees bent and your feet flat.

Steps:

1. Bring your left knee toward your chest as you flex your left foot. *a*

2. Straighten your left knee and move your foot as straight upward as you can, so that the sole of your left foot faces the ceiling. Hold this position briefly, feeling the stretch. *b*

3. Bend your left knee again, near your chest. *c*

4. Straighten your left knee in an outward motion this time, as though trying to kick something away from you. *d*

5. Bend your left knee. *e*

6. Straighten your left knee once more, close to the floor. *f*

7. Repeat these movements with your right knee.

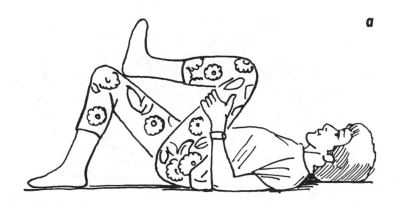

a

KNEE KICKS

Bending and straightening the knee at varying heights gives it a full stretch. You'll feel the pull in the big quadriceps muscle that runs through each thigh.

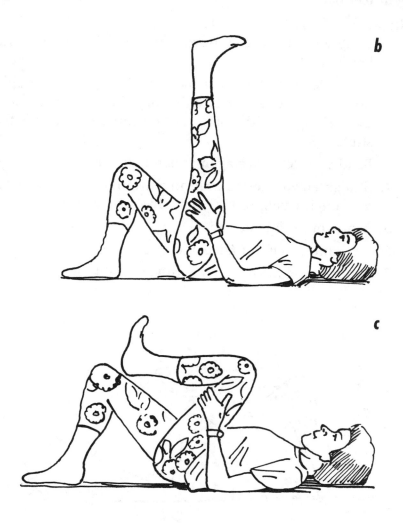

b

c

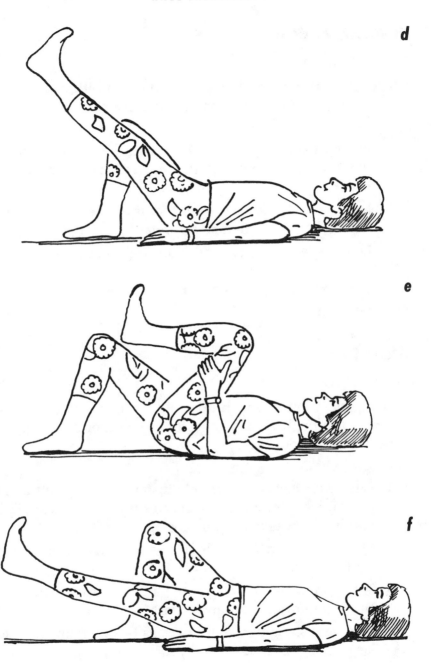

d

e

f

FORCED MARCH

Type: Stretching

Starting position: Stand in a comfortable position. You may use the back of a chair to lean on for support if need be.

Steps:

1. Bend and raise your left knee as high as you can, as though you were taking a step in an exaggerated military march.

2. Lower your left knee so your foot is on the floor where it started. (No need to march forward.)

3. Repeat the movement with your right knee.

Note: This exercise also appears in the section on Hips, as it benefits those joints as well.

BALLET BENDS

Type: Strengthening

Starting position: Stand comfortably with your feet apart. You may use the back of a chair for support, or simply place your hands on your hips.

Steps:

1. With your feet a comfortable distance apart and turned outward, bend your knees. Try to keep your back straight and your knees over your toes. *a*

2. Straighten your knees to lift your body back to the starting position.

3. Turn your feet so that they are parallel to each other, but still a comfortable distance apart. *b*

4. Bend and straighten your knees as before. Remember to keep your back straight and your knees pointing directly over your toes.

BALLET BENDS

These dancer's knee-bends are called pliés when done at the ballet barre. As you attempt them, remember to keep your knees directly over your toes.

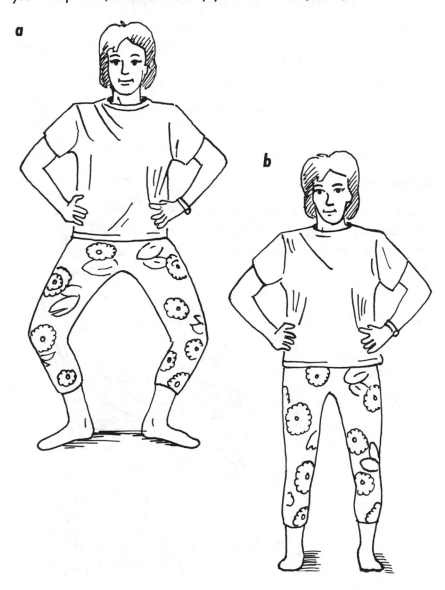

CHAIR BEND

Type: Stretching and strengthening

Starting position: Sit in a straight-back chair.

Steps:

1. Bend your left knee as far as you can, so that your foot moves under the chair.
2. Return to the starting position.
3. Repeat the movement with the right leg.

CHAIR BEND

Strengthen your knees by bending each one individually, as far as you can, so that you bring your foot up under you as you sit in a chair.

CANCAN

Type: Stretching

Starting position: Stand comfortably, giving yourself a chair or other sturdy support to lean on.

Steps:
1. Bend and raise your left knee.
2. With your dangling left foot, make small clockwise circles in the air.
3. Make counterclockwise circles with your left foot.
4. Return to the starting position.
5. Repeat the movements with your right knee and foot.

Note: This exercise also appears in the section on Hips, as it benefits those joints as well.

CHAIR LIFT

Type: Stretching and strengthening

Starting position: Sit in a straight-back chair with your feet flat on the floor.

Steps:
1. Lift your left foot out in front until your left knee is straight.
2. Slowly lower your left foot.
3. Repeat the movement with your right foot.

CHAIR LIFT, continued

Advanced addition: Position your chair in front of a coffee table or a footstool. When you extend your leg, rest your foot on this support. Straighten your knee as much as you can. Then, for added stretch, lean slightly forward from your waist, keeping your back straight. You will feel the stretch in the backs of your thighs—your hamstring muscles.

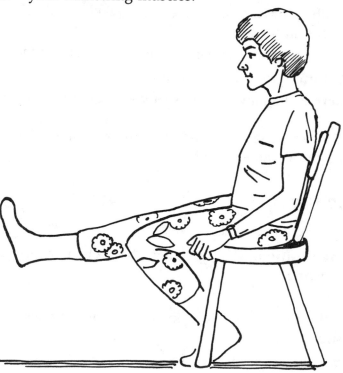

CHAIR LIFT

You can stretch and strengthen your knee by extending your leg straight out from a sitting position. Get the most extension you can, to keep your knee functioning at its best. For extra benefit, set your foot on a stool or coffee table. Then straighten your knee as much as you can and try to lean forward slightly.

166

SACK RACE

Type: Strengthening

Starting position: Sit in a straight-backed chair with an exercise belt looped around your ankles.

Steps:
1. Extend your left leg forward and your right leg back, pushing and pulling against the resistance of the belt.
2. Relax.
3. Reverse, so that you extend your right leg forward and pull your left leg back.

SACK RACE

An exercise belt or bungie cord will help strengthen your knees as you provide resistance by working one leg against the other.

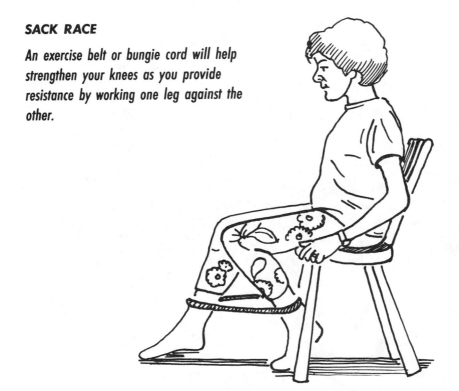

DIG YOUR HEELS IN

Type: Strengthening

Starting position: Sit in a straight-backed chair with your feet on the floor and the backs of your heels touching the front legs of the chair.

Steps:

1. Push back with your left foot as hard as you can, feeling the driving force in your knee.
2. Relax.
3. Repeat with the right foot.

CHAPTER 19

Exercises for the Ankles and Feet

How to use exercise to keep you on your toes

Bearing the full weight of the body, the large and small joints of the feet need exercise and comfortable shoes to keep them functioning well. Stretching and strengthening will also bolster the tendons and ligaments, making them less likely to succumb to sprains and other injuries.

These exercises include some fancy footwork from soft-shoe dance routines—that can be done while sitting down.

ANKLE TWIST

Type: Stretching

Starting position: Lie on your back with your legs extended and slightly apart.

Steps:

1. Rotate your ankles so that your feet point in, toward each other. Hold this position briefly. *a*

2. Rotate your ankles in the opposite direction, pointing your feet out. Hold briefly. *b*

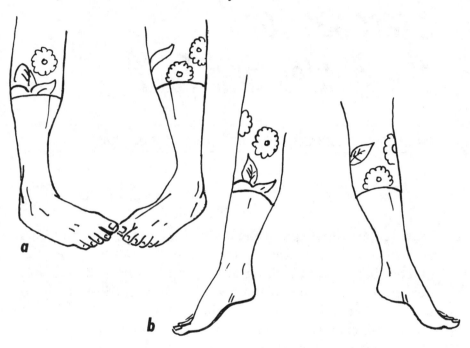

ANKLE TWIST

Bring your toes together, then apart, by moving just your ankles.

This is a smooth rotation movement that makes your feet work like slow-speed windshield wipers.

FOOT CIRCLES

Type: Stretching

Starting position: You may lie in bed with one foot hanging free over the edge of the mattress, or sit in a straight-back chair, raising one leg at a time to give each foot full freedom of movement.

Steps:
1. Circle your left foot in a clockwise direction.
2. Circle your left foot in a counterclockwise direction.
3. Repeat these movements with your right foot.

TOE CURLS

Type: Stretching

Starting position: You may lie down or sit in a straight-back chair.

Steps:
1. Curl your toes tightly.
2. Straighten and spread out your toes as far as you can.

TOE HELPER

Type: Gentle stretching and strengthening

Starting position: You may try this exercise while sitting or lying down.

Steps:
1. One at a time, put each toe through its full range of motion by moving it with your hand.
2. One at a time, try to exert pressure with each toe by pressing it against your fingers.

ANKLE STRETCH

Type: Stretching

Starting position: Sit in a straight-back chair with both feet flat on the floor.

Steps:
1. Raise your heels while you keep your toes on the floor.
2. Return to the starting position.
3. Raise your toes and arches, but leave your heels on the floor.

SOFT SHOE

Type: Stretching

Starting position: Sit in a straight-back chair with both feet flat on the floor.

Steps:
1. Raise your heels off the floor, as in the Ankle Stretch. *a*
2. Swivel both heels to the right before bringing them back down. Your feet are now pointing at an angle. *b*
3. Raise your toes and arches, leaving your heels on the floor.
4. Swivel the fronts of your feet to the right.
5. Repeat steps 1–4.
6. Raise your toes and arches, and swivel them to the left.
7. Raise your heels, and swivel them to the left.
8. Repeat steps 6 and 7—twice.
9. "Dance" back to the starting position.

SOFT SHOE

Use your ankles to swivel your feet, first on tiptoe, then on your heels. Tap dancers have incorporated this motion in many a dance routine.

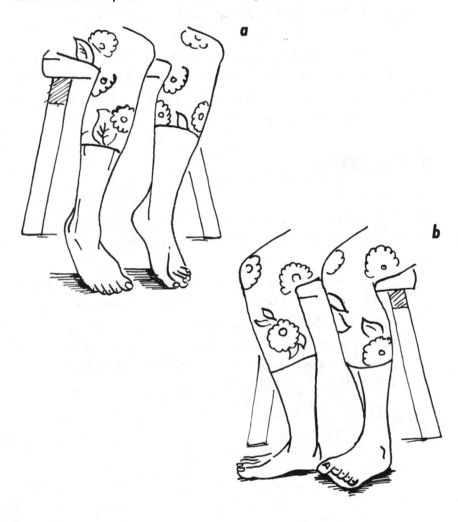

FOOT ROLL

Type: Stretching

Starting position: Sit in a straight-back chair. Place a rolling pin on the floor where you can reach it with your feet.

Steps:
1. Work the rolling pin with the bottoms of your feet to massage your arches and stretch your ligaments.
2. Work the rolling pin under your toes, curling and stretching them, too.

SIDE STRETCH

Type: Stretching

Starting position: Sit in a straight-back chair with your feet flat on the floor and your knees slightly apart.

Steps:
1. Rotate your ankles and lift your arches so that only the outer edges of your feet remain on the floor. *a*
2. Return to the starting position.
3. Rotate your ankles and lift the outer edges of your feet so that your knees come together and the big toes and inner heels stay on the floor. *b*

SIDE STRETCH

Lift your arches, but don't lift your feet off the floor, so that the soles of your feet face each other.

Put your feet back on the floor and then roll onto your arches. Your ankles should be doing all the work.

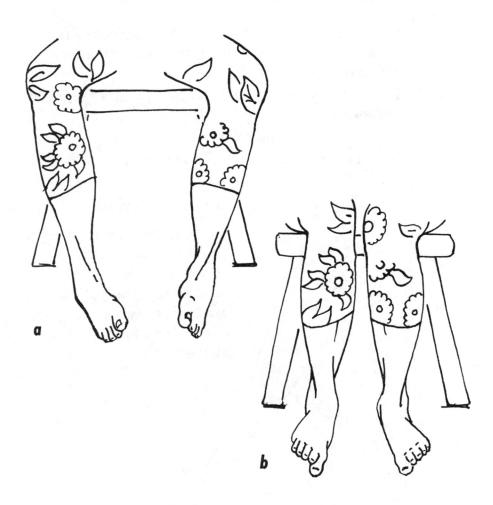

a

b

RUNNER'S STRETCH

Type: Stretching

Starting position: Stand facing a wall with your hands on the wall at about shoulder height and your feet a few inches from the wall base.

Steps:

1. Extend your left leg behind you, keeping your left knee straight, your toes on the floor, and your left heel raised. You may bend your right knee.
2. Try to lower your left heel to the floor, feeling the stretch in your Achilles tendon.
3. Return to the starting position.
4. Repeat the movements with your right leg.

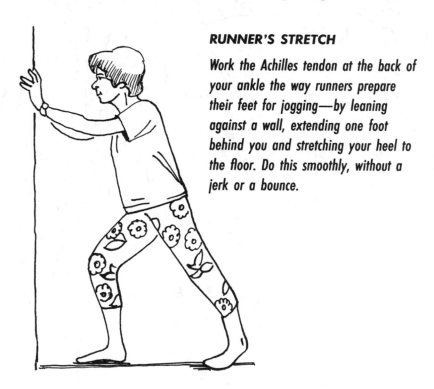

RUNNER'S STRETCH

Work the Achilles tendon at the back of your ankle the way runners prepare their feet for jogging—by leaning against a wall, extending one foot behind you and stretching your heel to the floor. Do this smoothly, without a jerk or a bounce.

ANKLE WALKOUT

Type: Stretching and strengthening

Starting position: Stand where you have room to walk.

Steps:

1. Walk a few paces on tiptoe. **a**
2. Walk a few paces on your heels. **b**

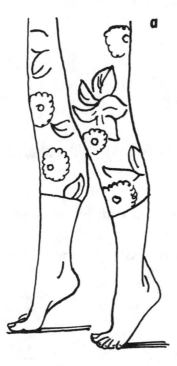

a

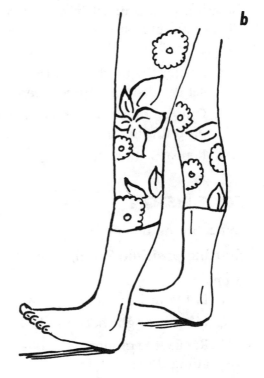

b

ANKLE WALKOUT

Throw your weight into this ankle exercise by walking first on tiptoe, then down on your heels. Keep a sturdy chair handy for balance and safety's sake.

ANKLE BUILDER

Type: Strengthening

Starting position: Stand, holding on to a sturdy support.

Steps:
1. Rise up on tiptoe.
2. Come down slowly.
3. Raise your toes so that you stand on your heels.
4. Put your feet flat on the floor.

STUNT WORK

Materials: Marbles, small dish or cup

Type: Strengthening

Starting position: Sit in a straight-back chair, with a small dish of marbles at your feet.

Steps:
1. Scatter the marbles on the floor, near your left foot, and set the dish or cup between your feet.
2. One by one, pick up each marble with your toes, and drop it into the dish.
3. Repeat with right foot.

FOOT PISTON

Type: Strengthening

Starting position: Stand, holding on to a sturdy support.

Steps:
1. Lift your left heel but leave your toes on the floor. *a*
2. Lift your right heel and lower your left. *b*
3. Repeat the motion, with one heel going up as the other is going down.

FOOT PISTON

As one heel goes up, the other one comes down.

Neither foot ever fully leaves the floor during this exercise, but the ankles keep pumping like pistons.

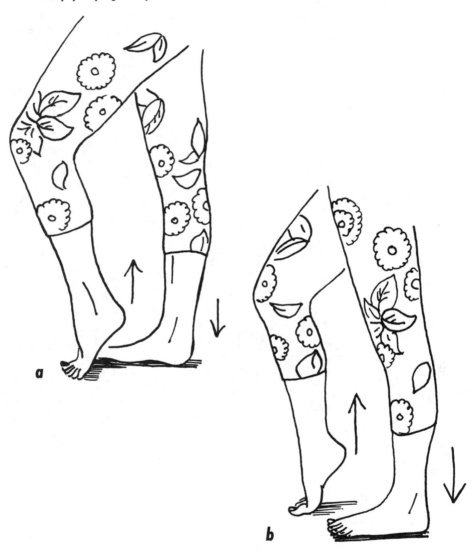

P A R T
F I V E

Exercising under Special Circumstances

> Since the activity of your arthritis
> may vary, your exercise program
> may vary as well. Do more when
> you're feeling well, less when
> you're not, but still do therapeutic
> exercises daily. . . . In addition, it
> is important to get in as good
> shape as possible in preparation for
> a time when you may not be able
> to exercise as actively as you
> would like.
>
> —Fred G. Kantrowitz, M.D.
> author, *Taking Control of Arthritis*

CHAPTER 20

When Flare-Ups Interfere

How to modify your arthritis exercise program while coping with a sudden, dramatic worsening of your symptoms

Anyone who exercises outdoors has to lose a day occasionally on account of bad weather, but people with arthritis can encounter bad days even in full sunshine. Sometimes, joint pain or swelling may increase for no apparent reason, necessitating a change in routine.

Rheumatoid arthritis is a disease that goes in cycles. If you have it, you've no doubt found that you can experience long periods of general well-being, when your pain is under control. Then, for no apparent reason, a "flare-up" will come along and aggravate your symptoms. You suffer from added pain and an increased number of stiff, swollen joints. You may even feel sick all over at these times—weak and feverish, so that you need to rest in bed.

People with osteoarthritis also recognize times when pain seems worse than usual, for reasons unknown.

Before you began exercising regularly, you may have reacted differently to flare-ups. You may have attributed them to the weather, to lack of sleep, a change in medication, or an increase in stress. Now the temptation may be to associate the flare-up with your exercise routine. You may have a whole new set of questions and concerns:

- Should I continue to exercise?
- What will happen if I exercise stiff or swollen joints?
- How can I balance rest and exercise during a flare-up?

First of all, we want to assure you that exercise itself does not cause a flare-up. Some people fear that their increased activity may have aggravated their arthritis, when in fact the opposite is true. Exercise improves the overall condition of your body. Flare-ups may occur in any case because the normal course of arthritis is erratic. Please don't blame yourself for your suffering!

During an arthritis flare-up, you may need to curtail aerobic exercise, but you don't have to stop exercising altogether. It isn't even advisable to do so. Most joints, including the inflamed ones, reap benefits from moving through their full range of motion once or twice a day. Should you find that this amount of gentle stretching is impossible because movement hurts too much, isometric strengthening exercises that involve no motion may still be performed to good advantage.

If your first thought at the onset of the flare-up was of abandoning your exercise program, we urge you to put that thought out of your mind. Concentrate instead on how to modify your exercise program during the current crisis—with an eye toward getting back in full swing as soon as you feel well enough to do so.

Aerobic Adjustments

Depending on the extent of the flare-up, you may have to abstain from your regular aerobic activities for a while. No doubt, you'll find that you miss your daily walk or swim. You miss the chance to get out and the energy boost that exercise always gives you. Try not to fret over this change, but simply recognize it and realize how important exercise has become in your life—and will be again!

You may also find that you feel depressed. Pain alone can bring on depression, but lack of exercise in a person conditioned to its benefits often produces a mild downward mood swing.

Your body will definitely respond to the change. Exercising is a little bit like eating, in that you have to keep doing it regularly to stay healthy. As soon as you stop exercising, you start losing the edge you've gained. Your muscle bulk gets smaller and the ability of your muscles to perform work decreases. In other words, when you get back to your routine, you'll need at least a few days to build up to your preflare-up level of fitness.

Stretching

You can continue to perform gentle range-of-motion exercises even while confined to your bed. Move every joint every day—except, of course, those in which pain seems to be exacerbated by movement.

If the flare-up has forced you to cut back on aerobic activity or cut it out altogether, by all means use the extra time you have to put your joints through their range of motion more frequently. By keeping up the stretching routines as best

185

you can, you help yourself maintain the progress you've made. You can't, of course, expect to greatly increase your flexibility during a flare-up.

Strengthening

Since your affected joints are exquisitely sensitive to motion during a flare-up, you may find the isotonic strengthening exercises—the ones that require you to move against an opposing force—too much of a strain. The isometrics, however, with their motionless, muscle-building pressure, may prove the perfect maneuvers for you at this time.

Isometrics can help you build strength in your wrists when you press the palms of your hands together, bolster your neck muscles when you press one palm against your forehead, improve your shoulder (or hip) condition when you work your arm (or leg) against a wall, strengthen your elbows when you push up from under a heavy table with your forearms, and brace your back by leaning hard against a chair-back or wall.

CHAPTER 21

Before and After Surgery

How to modify your exercise program to meet the
requirements for joint replacement or other surgical
procedures related to arthritis

Roughly one out of five members of our original Arthritis Survey group went through surgical procedures to find relief from arthritis pain. If you are currently facing an operation, you will discover, as they did, that exercise is a crucial element of both preoperative conditioning and postoperative healing.

As anxious as you may be about the procedure, remember that surgery for arthritis is among the most successful treatments for severe, intractable pain and disability. Rest assured that performing the right exercises will improve the likelihood of a good outcome in the long run.

Your specific exercise prescription will be dictated by the type of surgery you face. The most popular forms are:

- *Arthroplasty* to partially or totally replace or resurface a damaged joint, usually the hip or the knee
- *Arthrodesis* to fuse the bones of a joint in order to stabilize it, typically the ankle or the wrist
- *Arthroscopy*, or the use of fiber optics and miniature tools inserted through small incisions, to remove cartilage or other damaged tissue, most frequently in the knee.

Before

If you are suffering enough pain and joint deterioration to require surgery, you may have very limited movement in your affected joint. Indeed, you may be unable to perform any exercise other than isometric strengthening or passive stretching—letting your physical therapist carefully move the joint through its range of motion.

A muscle's natural state is motion, and enforced lack of motion will shrink the size of the tissue. Muscles may lose as much as thirty percent of their bulk in one week's worth of inactivity.

Your challenge during this preparation for the surgery period is to heed your body's pain messages while you get yourself in shape for the coming operation. On the one hand, you want to save the joint any unnecessary stress or pain. On the other hand, you want the rest of your body in tip-top condition for the combined stresses of anesthesia and prolonged rest. The more strength you amass before surgery, the speedier your recovery is likely to be.

We urge you to try to preserve your aerobic fitness as part of your preoperative preparation. If you're having surgery on your shoulders or hands, you may experience no difficulty sticking to your regular walking or cycling routine. But what if the surgery involves the weight-bearing joints of your hips or knees? Take heart—you can still find ways to work out. One solution is a hand-held bicycle called an arm-cycle ergometer, which should be available through the physical therapy department at your hospital. You'll find that you really have to spin the wheels with all your might to get the most out of this gadget, but it's probably worth the effort and definitely worth a try.

Such energy expenditure not only primes the heart and lungs, as you know, but can help you lose weight by burning calories and fat. If your upcoming surgery involves one of your weight-bearing joints, this may be the ideal time to try to shed extra pounds. Why give the weight-bearing joints any excess weight to bear?

The impending surgery may give you the incentive you've been lacking to do something about your weight. But don't opt for a crash diet that could leave you weakened by lack of important nutrients. You need your strength for surgery. You'll do best if you combine your aerobic exercise with a healthful diet, high in fiber but low in fat and calories.

As a safety precaution, you will be asked to drop your usual medications before surgery. If you take aspirin, your doctor will ask you to do without it beginning about two weeks prior to your operation. The reason is that aspirin interferes with blood clotting, and taking it could lead to unnecessary bleeding. One week before surgery, you will be asked to drop any other anti-inflammatory drugs you've been taking, for the same reason. (Your doctor may suggest that you rely on acetaminophen instead, best known by its brand name Tylenol, as this drug has no apparent influence on blood clotting.)

Any change in your regular medications may lead to a temporary increase in pain and may make it more difficult for you to exercise. As usual, it makes sense to heed the pain messages. Don't force your body to follow your regular exercise regimen under these circumstances. You'll get back to a full program soon—and then some.

After

A physical therapist may be your first visitor after surgery. Indeed, the exercises you will be doing for rehabilitation are every bit as important as the surgery you went through. One cannot succeed without the other.

The exercise apparatus the therapist brings you for the start of your postoperative exercise program could be anything from a handful of therapeutic putty to squeeze with your new finger joints to a machine that will flex and straighten your new knee as though you were riding an automatic bicycle. The therapist will supervise you at first, and direct you as to how you should increase your activity as you grow stronger.

Try not to be discouraged if you discover that you feel less fit and have a narrower range of motion than you did beforehand. Remember how much time you've needed to rest, and that inactivity causes weakness. Slowly and steadily, you can regain the ground you've lost if you just keep up with your modified exercise regimen.

Among your cheeriest thoughts will be the realization that your pain in the affected joint has decreased dramatically or disappeared altogether. You may feel wobbly and out of sorts at first, but freedom from pain will enable you to pursue your rehabilitation program and return to full activity.

Find out from your doctor precisely what you can and cannot do during your recovery period. Make sure you understand how much time you will have to allow for full recovery. The surgery you've had should lead eventually to greater mobility and independence, but for right now, give yourself every chance to achieve the best possible long-term outcome by doing less than ever. Your family and friends will no doubt want to help you shop, cook, and do other errands and chores. Let them.

If you have received an artificial joint, be sure to ask about any special restrictions that may apply to it. Ask your doctor and your physical therapist. Either one may tell you things the other forgets to mention. In the first few weeks of living with a new hip joint, for example, one has to be careful not to disturb the replacement by bending too much. Observe these precautions to guarantee yourself the longest possible life for your artificial joint.

CHAPTER 22

While Coping with Other Health Problems

How to balance an arthritis exercise program with the special demands created by other illnesses and medications

People with arthritis are not immune to other widespread health problems such as heart disease, high blood pressure, and diabetes.

Sometimes the coincidence of arthritis with another illness in the same body is just a run of bad luck. In many cases, however, arthritis medications may actually be the cause of the second condition. Ulcers, for example, are an all-too-frequent side effect of taking high doses of aspirin or other anti-inflammatory drugs. High blood pressure may develop with the fluid retention that often results from treatment with corticosteroids such as prednisone.* Diabetes may also follow in the wake of steroid drug use, and osteoporosis is yet another potential complication.

Proper exercise with proper precautions can benefit any or all of these conditions. As a person with two or more health issues to consider, you'll want to pick and choose your exercises with extra care.

The range-of-motion exercises you do for your arthritic joints are so gentle as to pose no risk to other body systems. Strengthening exercises, however, especially the isometric ones, are a different matter. Even though these muscle builders involve no motion, and are therefore painless enough to perform even during an arthritis flare-up, they may pose special problems for people with heart disease and high blood pressure. If you have either of these conditions, you will need your doctor's approval before attempting isometrics as they can cause brief interruptions in blood circulation.

Aerobic exercise is recommended across the board, as it has so much to offer. We've already ticked off the many advantages, including strength, flexibility, pain reduction, weight control, longevity, and a general feeling of well-being. In arthritis care, aerobic exercise helps preserve joint motion and prevent joint deformity. Let's look at its specific advantages in addressing other health problems.

Heart Disease

If you suffer from heart disease, aerobic exercise can help you strengthen the heart muscle itself. Aerobic exercise first became a household word for this proven positive effect on the

---

*Other corticosteroids prescribed for our original Arthritis Survey group of 1,051 participants include cortisone acetate, methylprednisolone, dexamethasone, prednisolone, and triamcinolone.

heart. Indeed, it is often called cardiovascular exercise because it improves the function of the whole circulatory system.

The cardiologist who treats you for heart disease will want to have a say in your exercise program, and will determine how much of a workout is safe for you by means of an exercise treadmill test (see page 196). Without question, the prescribed activity will be walking. As Dr. Dean Ornish explains in his book, *Reversing Heart Disease*, walking is the preferred form of exercise because it provides the most health benefits and poses the lowest risk of injury or sudden cardiac arrest.

Dr. Ornish counsels the patients in his "Opening Your Heart" program to walk at least thirty minutes every day, or one hour three times a week. If you have advanced arthritis in your weight-bearing joints, you may not be able to walk this much, at least not when you first start to exercise. But it's nice to know that you can stride for stronger legs and improve your heart's health while you do so.

We have not, up to now, discussed target heart rates or metabolic equivalent units—two subjects that pepper the conversation of exercise enthusiasts. Our reason? We merely want you to move, to find relief from pain, to gain flexibility, to extend the range of motion in your joints, and to discover pleasure in aerobic activity. We're not urging you to become a fitness freak or a marathon runner.

Now, however, in a discussion of heart problems, target heart rate becomes relevant.* In brief, you serve your heart best by exercising in a sustained fashion that makes your heart pump faster than when you're sitting still. The ideal, or target

---

*Metabolic equivalent units, or METs, offer another way to measure the intensity with which you exercise. METs are expressed in amounts of energy used for energy production, per minute. You use one MET just sitting still. If your maximum MET value is 6, then your body consumes six times as much oxygen going at full tilt than it uses at rest.

rate, is between forty-five and eighty percent of your heart's top speed. As you can imagine, pushing to the limit poses dangers, which is why doctors like to determine that limit in a controlled setting, where they can take care of you right away if something goes wrong. The exercise treadmill test, or an exercise cycle test, performed in a hospital or doctor's office, with electrocardiogram and blood pressure monitoring, meets all these conditions.

Once you've been informed of your target heart rate, you can easily determine, during your exercise sessions, whether you're pushing your heart hard enough. Simply place the flat of your fingertip on the inside of your wrist, near the base of your thumb, where you can feel your blood pulsing through the radial artery. Using a watch with a second hand, count how many beats you feel in a ten-second period. Then you can multiply the result by six to find your heart rate (pulse). Or, you can start with the target range and divide those numbers by six, so you know what your ten-second pulse should be.

The medications you take for your heart condition will no doubt influence the way you respond to exercise. Beta blockers (such as Inderal, Lopressor, and Tenormin) tend to slow down the heart rate and lower the blood pressure—just the way exercise does over time. Nitrates (including Nitro-Bid and Nitro-Dur), on the other hand, speed up the heart rate while they lower the blood pressure. By keeping your doctor informed of your exercise progress, you'll be able to make any needed adjustments in drug dosage as your body becomes more fit.

Hypertension

If hypertension, or high blood pressure, is your problem, you may well be wondering what all the increased blood flow promised by exercise will mean for you. Won't your blood pressure rise even higher? The fact is, while your blood pressure may increase temporarily during an exercise session, it will drop to a lower level as a result of regular exercise. And the weight loss you may experience from all that brisk walking will help lower it even further.

By all means, check with your doctor about your exercise plans. It may turn out that you can decrease or even drop the medications you take for your high blood pressure once exercise becomes a regular habit.

Diabetes

Whether your diabetes traces from childhood or became a problem only recently, exercise offers one way to gain control over your blood sugar—with your doctor's advice and consent.

Like insulin, physical activity takes up blood sugar. This means that regular exercise will most likely change the amount of insulin you need to take. In fact, some people with Type II (adult onset) diabetes may reach a point where they no longer require any medication. Exercise and diet alone may provide all the necessary regulation of their blood sugar levels.

When you begin your exercise program, take careful note of your blood sugar at the start of each activity period, and again at the end. See whether you need to modify your insulin dosage, and discuss the changes with your doctor.

It's a good idea to time your exercise according to your insulin schedule to avoid problems. If, for example, you set out for a brisk walk during the peak of your insulin response, you may suddenly feel weak and dizzy due to hypoglycemia. Be assured that you can find a way to coordinate your exercise prescription with your medicine prescriptions—it just takes a little time and careful consideration.

ABOUT THE

AUTHORS

Dava Sobel and Arthur C. Klein are the authors of *Arthritis: What Works* (St. Martin's Press 1989, 1990, 1992), an evaluation of treatments that really help, based on an unprecedented nationwide Arthritis Survey™ of 1,051 participants with osteo- or rheumatoid arthritis. *Arthritis: What Works* has sold nearly half a million copies, and was chosen as a selection of the Prevention Book Club. The authors' first book, *Backache Relief* (Times Books 1985, NAL/Signet 1986), a Book-of-the-Month Club alternate selection, grew out of a survey of 500 back pain sufferers from all 50 states, and exposed the startling truth about the best sources of care and the most effective treatments.

Having completed this special volume on arthritis exercise, the authors are at work on a new book about back exercise.

The authors would love to hear about your experiences with exercise for arthritis. You can write to them with comments or questions about the program outlined here—or to share

199

specific exercises that have been helpful to you, for possible inclusion in a future edition of this book. Please address your letters to:

> Dava Sobel and Arthur C. Klein
> c/o Arthritis Survey™
> St. Martin's Press, Inc., Box JTK
> 175 Fifth Avenue
> New York, NY 10010

John H. Bland, M.D., is a professor of medicine at the University of Vermont College of Medicine in Burlington. He teaches, practices, and conducts research in rheumatology— the field of medicine that concerns arthritis and related diseases. Internationally recognized as an authority in his field, Dr. Bland was named a Master of Rheumatology by the American College of Rheumatology. He is a fellow of the American College of Physicians and the American College of Sports Medicine.

His research has been supported by the National Institutes of Health and the Arthritis Foundation. The author of several books and many journal articles, Dr. Bland also serves on the editorial board of the Journal of Rheumatology.